THE BEST
IN TENT
CAMPING

NEW JERSEY

D1413360

Other titles in the series:

The Best in Tent Camping: The Carolinas
The Best in Tent Camping: Colorado
The Best in Tent Camping: Florida
The Best in Camping: Georgia
The Best in Tent Camping: Minnesota
The Best in Tent Camping: Missouri and the Ozarks
The Best in Tent Camping: Montana
The Best in Tent Camping: New England
The Best in Tent Camping: Northern California
The Best in Tent Camping: Oregon
The Best in Tent Camping: The Southern Appalachian and Smoky Mountains
The Best in Tent Camping: Southern California
The Best in Tent Camping: Tennessee and Kentucky
The Best in Tent Camping: Virginia
The Best in Camping: Washington
The Best in Tent Camping: West Virginia
The Best in Tent Camping: Wisconsin

THE BEST IN TENT CAMPING

A GUIDE FOR CAR CAMPERS WHO HATE RVs,
CONCRETE SLABS, AND LOUD PORTABLE STEREOS

NEW JERSEY

MARIE JAVINS

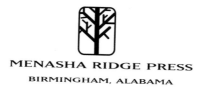

MENASHA RIDGE PRESS
BIRMINGHAM, ALABAMA

*For fellow 8th Street freelancers Roberta Melzl and Yancey Labat,
who regularly reminded me that there is life beyond the laptop.
Thanks for the distractions and understanding.*

Copyright © 2005 Marie Javins
All rights reserved
Printed in the United States of America
Published by Menasha Ridge Press
Distributed by the Globe Pequot Press
First edition, first printing

Library of Congress Cataloging in Publication
Javins, Marie
    The best in tent camping, New Jersey: a guide for car campers who hate RVs, concrete
    slabs, and loud portable stereos / by Marie Javins.—1st. ed.
    p. cm.
    Includes bibliographical references and index.
    ISBN 0-89732-596-6

    1. Camp sites, facilities, etc.—New Jersey—Guidebooks. 2. Camping—New Jersey—
    Guidebooks. 3. New Jersey—Guidebooks. I. Title.

GV191.42.N5J38 2005
917.49'068—dc22   2005041677

Cover and text design by Ian Szymkowiak, Palace Press International, Inc.
Cover photo by Susan E. Degginger/Alamy
Maps by Bryan Steven Jones

Menasha Ridge Press
P.O. Box 43673
Birmingham, Alabama 35243
www.menasharidge.com

TABLE OF CONTENTS

STATE MAPS KEY vii
NEW JERSEY CAMPGROUND LOCATOR MAP viii
ACKNOWLEDGMENTS x
PREFACE xi
MAP LEGEND xii
INTRODUCTION 2

NORTHERN NEW JERSEY
CAMPGAW MOUNTAIN 8
CAMP GLEN GRAY 11
RAMAPO VALLEY COUNTY RESERVATION 14
WEIS ECOLOGY CENTER 17

WESTERN NEW JERSEY
CAMP TAYLOR 22
DELAWARE WATER GAP NATIONAL RECREATION AREA (CANOE-IN) 25
DELAWARE WATER GAP NATIONAL RECREATION AREA/APPALACHIAN TRAIL (HIKE-IN) 28
HARMONY RIDGE CAMPGROUND 31
HIGH POINT STATE PARK 34
JENNY JUMP STATE FOREST 37
MAHLON DICKERSON RESERVATION 40
STEPHENS STATE PARK 43
STOKES STATE FOREST LAKE OCQUITTUNK CAMPING AREA 46
STOKES STATE FOREST SHOTWELL CAMPING AREA 49
STOKES STATE FOREST STEAM MILL CAMPING AREA 52
SWARTSWOOD STATE PARK 55
WORTHINGTON STATE FOREST 58

CENTRAL NEW JERSEY
ALLAIRE STATE PARK 62
BULL'S ISLAND RECREATION AREA 65
CHEESEQUAKE STATE PARK 68
DELAWARE RIVER FAMILY CAMPGROUND 71
ROUND VALLEY RECREATION AREA 74
SPRUCE RUN RECREATION AREA 77
TEETERTOWN RAVINE NATURE PRESERVE 80
TRIPLE BROOK CAMPING RESORT 83

TURKEY SWAMP PARK 86
VOORHEES STATE PARK 89

THE JERSEY SHORE
ATLANTIC CITY NORTH FAMILY CAMPGROUND 94
BASS RIVER STATE FOREST 97
BIRCH GROVE PARK 100
CEDAR CREEK CAMPGROUND 103
NORTH WILDWOOD CAMPING RESORT 106
RIVERWOOD PARK 109
SURF AND STREAM CAMPGROUND 112
TIMBERLINE LAKE CAMPING RESORT 115

SOUTHERN NEW JERSEY
ATLANTIC COUNTY PARK AT ESTELL MANOR 120
ATLANTIC COUNTY PARK AT LAKE LENAPE 123
BELLEPLAIN STATE FOREST MEISLE FIELD AND CCC CAMP 126
BELLEPLAIN STATE FOREST NORTHSHORE CAMPGROUND 129
BRENDAN T. BYRNE STATE FOREST 132
FRONTIER CAMPGROUND 135
PARVIN STATE PARK 138
TIMBERLANE CAMPGROUND 141
WHARTON STATE FOREST: ATSION 144
WHARTON STATE FOREST: BATONA 147
WHARTON STATE FOREST: BODINE FIELD 150
WHARTON STATE FOREST: BUTTONWOOD HILL CAMP 153
WHARTON STATE FOREST: GODFREY BRIDGE CAMPING AREA 156
WHARTON STATE FOREST: GOSHEN POND CAMPING AREA 159
WHARTON STATE FOREST: LOWER FORGE AND MULLICA RIVER CAMPS 162

APPENDIXES
APPENDIX A—CAMPING EQUIPMENT CHECKLIST 167
APPENDIX B—SOURCES OF INFORMATION 169
APPENDIX C—SUGGESTED READING AND REFERENCE 171
INDEX 173

ABOUT THE AUTHOR 178

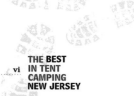

NEW JERSEY MAPS KEY

NORTHERN NEW JERSEY

1 CAMPGAW MOUNTAIN
2 CAMP GLEN GRAY
3 RAMAPO VALLEY COUNTY RESERVATION
4 WEIS ECOLOGY CENTER

WESTERN NEW JERSEY

5 CAMP TAYLOR
6 DELAWARE WATER GAP NATIONAL RECREATION AREA (CANOE-IN)
7 DELAWARE WATER GAP NATIONAL RECREATION AREA/APPALACHIAN TRAIL (HIKE-IN)
8 HARMONY RIDGE CAMPGROUND
9 HIGH POINT STATE PARK
10 JENNY JUMP STATE FOREST
11 MAHLON DICKERSON RESERVATION
12 STEPHENS STATE PARK
13 STOKES STATE FOREST LAKE OCQUITTUNK CAMPING AREA
14 STOKES STATE FOREST SHOTWELL CAMPING AREA
15 STOKES STATE FOREST STEAM MILL CAMPING AREA
16 SWARTSWOOD STATE PARK
17 WORTHINGTON STATE FOREST

CENTRAL NEW JERSEY

18 ALLAIRE STATE PARK
19 BULL'S ISLAND RECREATION AREA
20 CHEESEQUAKE STATE PARK
21 DELAWARE RIVER FAMILY CAMPGROUND
22 ROUND VALLEY RECREATION AREA
23 SPRUCE RUN RECREATION AREA
24 TEETERTOWN RAVINE NATURE PRESERVE
25 TRIPLE BROOK CAMPING RESORT

26 TURKEY SWAMP PARK
27 VOORHEES STATE PARK

THE JERSEY SHORE

28 ATLANTIC CITY NORTH FAMILY CAMPGROUND
29 BASS RIVER STATE FOREST
30 BIRCH GROVE PARK
31 CEDAR CREEK CAMPGROUND
32 NORTH WILDWOOD CAMPING RESORT
33 RIVERWOOD PARK
34 SURF AND STREAM CAMPGROUND
35 TIMBERLINE LAKE CAMPING RESORT

SOUTHERN NEW JERSEY

36 ATLANTIC COUNTY PARK AT ESTELL MANOR
37 ATLANTIC COUNTY PARK AT LAKE LENAPE
38 BELLEPLAIN STATE FOREST MEISLE FIELD AND CCC CAMP
39 BELLEPLAIN STATE FOREST NORTHSHORE CAMPGROUND
40 BRENDAN T. BYRNE STATE FOREST
41 FRONTIER CAMPGROUND
42 PARVIN STATE PARK
43 TIMBERLANE CAMPGROUND
44 WHARTON STATE FOREST: ATSION
45 WHARTON STATE FOREST: BATONA
46 WHARTON STATE FOREST: BODINE FIELD
47 WHARTON STATE FOREST: BUTTONWOOD HILL CAMP
48 WHARTON STATE FOREST: GODFREY BRIDGE CAMPING AREA
49 WHARTON STATE FOREST: GOSHEN POND CAMPING AREA
50 WHARTON STATE FOREST: LOWER FORGE AND MULLICA RIVER CAMPS

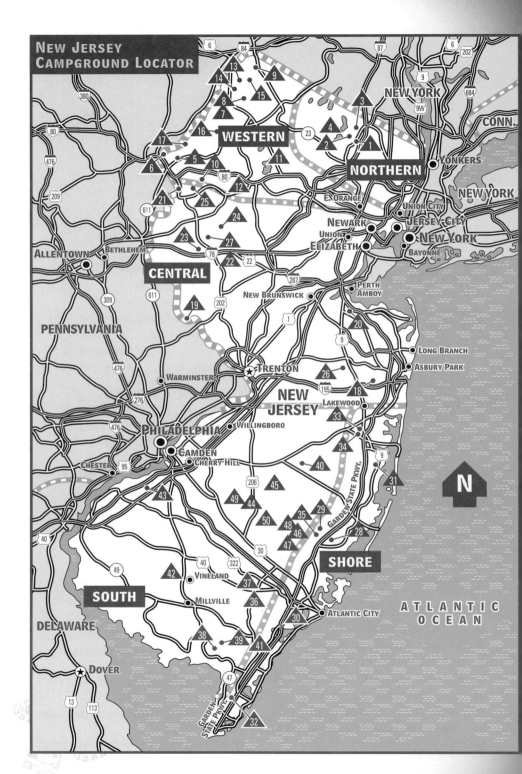

MAP LEGEND

WHITE WOLF

Campground name
and location

Individual tent and RV
campsites within
campground area

Table Rock

Other nearby
campgrounds

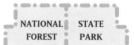
| NATIONAL FOREST | STATE PARK |
Public lands

Interstate
highways

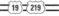
US
highways

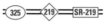
State   County   Service
roads   roads   roads

MAIN ST.
_____
Other roads

Unpaved or
gravel roads

Boardwalk

Political
boundary

+++++++
Railroads

- - - - -
Hiking, biking,
or horse trail

Swift Creek
River or stream

Asheville
◉
City
or town

N
Indicates North

Ward Lake
Ocean, lake,
or bay

Bridge or tunnel	Playground	Picnic area	
Amphitheater	Parking	Sheltered picnic area	
Falls or rapids	Marina or boat ramp	Spring/well	
Food	Fire ring	Dishwater disposal	
Restroom	Telephone	Summit or lookout	
Water access	Laundry	Bathhouse	
Gate	Cemetery	Dump station	
Trash	Swimming	No swimming	
Wheelchair accessible	Horse trail	Stables	
Hospital/medical care	Postal dropoff	Ranger office	

ACKNOWLEDGMENTS

THE COMPLETION OF THIS BOOK was aided by assistance from the following individuals: Michele Stelle of New Jersey State Park Service, Karla Risdon of Weis Ecology Center, Greg Vizzi of Atlantic County Parks, and Ramon of New York–New Jersey Trail Conference. Luis C. Pi-Sunyer of Camp Glen Gray and John Trontis of Hunterdon County Parks were especially helpful.

Special thanks to Mopsy Gascon for patient editing and prompt responses. Thanks to Russell Helms for not laughing at the idea of a book on tent camping in a state that is easily the most (unfairly) joked about state in the nation. Kudos to my family, friends, and other employers for putting up with me during the epic production of this book, and to my usually reliable old car for not breaking down until the very end of the project.

THE BEST IN TENT CAMPING

NEW JERSEY

PREFACE

BENJAMIN FRANKLIN IS CREDITED with having invented the Jersey joke. He supposedly referred to the Garden State as "a barrel tapped at both ends." This metaphor was not inaccurate—picture thousands of commuters pouring from the country's most densely populated state into Manhattan and Philadelphia—but it did start a long, undeserved tradition.

The Jersey joke outlasted the founding fathers, perpetuated by folks whose knowledge of the state was limited to knowing which exit of the New Jersey Turnpike took them off the highway (and out of the state) that they viewed as a necessary evil in their journey from "here" to "there."

But those who have seen only the much-maligned New Jersey Turnpike know just a tiny part of the state. They leave thinking that New Jersey is about massive rest areas, full-service gas stations, cargo ports, and roadside oil refineries. They laugh at the nickname "Garden State" and mock the exits that have efficiently delivered them to their destinations.

When I suggested a New Jersey camping guidebook to my editor at Menasha Ridge Press, I expected him to laugh and make a tired joke about camping amid toxic waste. Instead, I was asked to research the topic further. It didn't take long for me to report back that New Jersey was home to dozens of state and county parks and forests, the Pinelands National Reserve, two national recreation areas, scenic rivers, and 73.6 miles of the Appalachian Trail. Somehow, in spite of New Jersey's industrial past and populous present, the state has managed to protect more than 230,000 acres of state forest and 1.1 million acres of Pine Barrens. Not bad for the fourth-smallest state in the nation.

Camping under the stars along the Delaware River or beneath the Pine Barrens is a New Jersey experience not to be missed. You can relax alone in the most remote wilderness sites or you can enjoy the conveniences of developed campgrounds, where your neighbors may be behind the nearest hedge, but so is the bathhouse with the hot water and washing machine. Jersey's camping options rival the best in the country, but the dozens of quirky characteristics of the state make a visit to this state unique. New Jersey features plenty of urban legends, historic moments, and all-around wackiness that add to its charm. Where else can you hike the Appalachian Trail, visit a wolf preserve, view the birthplace of Frank Sinatra, and have a quick swim near the site of the 1916 shark attacks that inspired "Jaws," all before setting up camp in time for dinner?

But don't take my word for it. Arm yourself with one of the half-dozen guides to quirky sites in New Jersey, this guidebook, and some trail maps, and head out to the great outdoors. There's a lot of New Jersey beyond the Turnpike.

—*Marie Javins*

INTRODUCTION

WELCOME TO THE WESTERN MOUNTAINS and sandy pine forests of New Jersey, where you will unexpectedly find beautiful campgrounds that rival any in America. This is a densely populated state, with the vast majority of people crammed into the urban northeast and the cities, but it is also a small state. You are never more than a few hours from the Atlantic Ocean, the Appalachian Trail, or the solitude of the Pinelands. Whether you enjoy fishing, surfing, mountain biking, canoeing, or just staring at the stars from a remote campsite, New Jersey will surprise you with its state forests, public parks, and the occasional private-but-wooded campground. Even the most crowded areas feature parks, wetlands, wild raptors, and bike trails. Have the last laugh at all the Jersey jokesters and enjoy hundreds of miles of trails and rivers just around the corner from Manhattan or Philadelphia.

New Jersey has unique features that may appeal to more than the outdoors-oriented members of the family. To many, camping is about relaxing in serene wilderness, but to others it is an economic choice that offers affordable accommodation. Travelers bound for Philadelphia on a budget should check out Timberlane Campground, while visitors en route to Manhattan will want to focus on the campgrounds profiled in the "Northern" chapter. Beach and casino lovers should turn first to the "Shore" profiles.

Those looking for more natural environments where they can hike, canoe, and bike through the woods have the most choices. Every chapter describes vast parks and rivers waiting to be explored. The western side of the state features canoe-in sites along the Delaware River and hike-in sites along the Appalachian Trail. Campgrounds in southern New Jersey sit under the tall trees of the Pinelands National Reserve, which includes miles of forest and winding streams. Central New Jersey offers a campground for every interest, from the historic village of Allaire State Park to the bike and canoe trails that run through Bull's Island Recreation Area. Even northern New Jersey offers pockets of woodlands and outdoors educational centers.

One advantage of camping in such a small, developed state is that you are never far from businesses and stores. Even though your tent may be the only one in sight, with a few frogs or deer as your only companions, you can still easily rent a canoe or go for a swim in a lake with a lifeguard on duty. So grab your tent and head outside to the Garden State, home to mountains, rivers, forests, beaches, and excellent campgrounds.

THE RATING SYSTEM

Certain attributes are common to all New Jersey campgrounds and have been rated here using a star system. Five-star ratings are fantastic, while one star is acceptable. Ratings are subjective, but the star system can help campers identify their ideal campgrounds at a glance.

BEAUTY
In the wilds of the northwest, the most beautiful campgrounds sit among protected forests, their beauty obvious to tent campers who value thick greenery, craggy mountains, and the presence of wild animals. But beauty in the southern forest is defined differently, with the Pinelands' scrubby underbrush, cranberry bogs, and sandy ground—features that combine to make an ecosystem that is unique in the world. The beauty of the Pinelands reveals itself after the surprise at the environmental shift wears off.

PRIVACY
For those who seek wooded solitude, few campgrounds have sites far enough apart. Some campgrounds offer wide-open spaces as buffer zones, while others use natural barriers such as hedges and undergrowth to provide the illusion of privacy. In general, public campgrounds offer more seclusion than private campgrounds. Those who truly wish to be alone should seek out the wilderness camping areas listed in this book, where campers often have entire campgrounds to themselves.

SPACIOUSNESS
Not everyone is looking for a green clearing carved out of undergrowth and hardwoods. Some campers have large families, while others simply need space to park a boat or set up a kitchen tent. Family groups frequently visit the most popular New Jersey state parks, which may feature expansive adjacent sites. Specify the sort of site you prefer when reserving.

QUIET
No site in New Jersey is truly quiet, as birds, frogs, and insects can make quite a racket around camp. In New Jersey, you're never that far from a main thoroughfare, but campgrounds are cleverly designed so that sites are deep within parks, where the only non-natural noises might come from canoe paddles breaking the water or from cyclists whizzing by. To enhance the quiet of your natural setting, avoid summer weekend camping and set up camp midweek. The quietest sites are found in wilderness camping areas, which usually involve a hike in and out.

SECURITY
Remote, primitive sites feel safer than populated parklands. After all, who would hike 3 miles to steal a can of propane? But in more populated campgrounds, other campers will probably notice if a stranger is poking around your tent, and rangers patrol the area. Though campsite thievery is not likely to occur in remote or populated sites in New Jersey, common sense should still guide you. Leave valuables at home and pack tempting items into your car's trunk. The most likely thieves are the ones wearing fur and walking on four legs, and they are after your food. Leave all food and coolers in your trunk or in bear-proof containers.

CLEANLINESS

Many of New Jersey's state parks offer garbage bags at contact stations, and visitors are encouraged to carry out everything they carried in. Dumpsters are usually located near bathhouses, with allowances made for bear-proofing. Nevertheless, rubbish can accumulate after busy weekends. Popular parks are cleaned quickly, so busy does not necessarily equal dirty. Remote site are less fastidiously maintained, but rubbish is often organic, simply a byproduct of the elements acting in accord with nature. A low rating should not discourage you from visiting a campground—often the lower the cleanliness rating, the wilder the site.

A FEW WORDS ABOUT CRITTERS

Pets   New Jersey state parks do not allow pets in camping areas, so when traveling with a dog, campers are limited to regional or private sites in New Jersey.

Bears   Remember, New Jersey has an overpopulation of black bears. Black bears generally avoid humans, but many associate humans with food and have lost their fear of people. Do not keep food in your tent and do not cook anywhere near your tent. Take a bear-proof (and rodent-proof) container for your food. When not in use, keep your food locked in your car to avoid accidental conditioning of animals. Coolers must never leave the car and should be covered along with all food. Don't bury or burn garbage as bears will dig it up. Also, don't keep smelly items such as deodorant or soap in your tent. Bears are much nicer to look at from a distance than from across a small patch of canvas. If you break these rules, you will not only put yourself in danger, you will also be doing a disservice to the bear that may become accustomed to associating humans with food, turning into a "nuisance bear." Bears that cannot be reconditioned must be destroyed. Save a bear by following the rules.

If you should have an unexpected black bear encounter, stay upright and back away slowly. Speak in a calm voice. If you spot one as you hike, stay far away from it and make enough noise so that it is aware of your presence. Do not surprise the bear. Never get between a mother bear and her cub, and remember that while they may not be afraid of people, they are unpredictable wild animals. After an encounter, always contact the forest office so that rangers can drive over and use proper conditioning on the bear.

Snakes   Snakes, like bears, tend to appear when you least expect them. They like warm—but not hot—weather, and are active from mid-spring through mid-autumn. Most encounters with such reptiles involve benign garter snakes, rat snakes, ribbon snakes, and black racers. Venomous rattlesnakes and copperheads are also native to this area but are rarely seen. In general, their heads are more triangular than their nonvenomous cousins. You might spend a few minutes studying snakes before heading into the woods, but in any case, a good rule of thumb is to give whatever animal you encounter a wide berth and leave it alone.

Ticks   Ticks tend to lurk in the brush, leaves, and grass that grow alongside trails. April through mid-July is the peak period for ticks in this area, but it is possible to pick up stray ticks in every month of the year. Scientifically, ticks are arachnids (of the spider family) and ectoparasites, which live on the outside of a host for the majority of their life cycle in order to reproduce. Of the two varieties that may hitch a ride on you while hiking—wood ticks and deer ticks—extensive research suggests that both need several hours of actual bloodsucking attachment before they can transmit any disease. Deer ticks, the primary vector for Lyme disease, are very small (often as tiny as a poppy seed), and you may not be aware of their presence until you feel the itchiness of their bite. The best avoidance strategy is to wear light-colored clothing (so that you can spot the ticks more easily); tuck the bottom of your pant legs into your socks (sure it looks geeky, but it helps); lather your ankles, wrists, and neck with a DEET-rich insect repellant; and remain on the beaten path. At the end of the hike, check yourself thoroughly before getting in the car, bus, or train; and later, when you take a post-hike shower, do an even more thorough check of your entire body. Ticks that haven't bitten you are easily removed, but not easily killed, unless you burn or crush them. Tweezers work best for plucking off attached ticks.

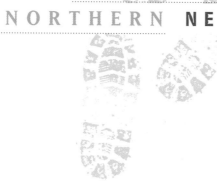

NORTHERN NEW JERSEY

CAMPGAW MOUNTAIN

FAMED FOR ITS SKI RESORT rather than its camping, Campgaw Mountain County Reservation takes a lot of heat in winter. Detractors are quick to point out that the trails are easy and the slopes are mild. Supporters defend Campgaw with stories of learning to ski there, in a friendly environment that enabled them to discover confidence in snow and the outdoors. Families take their children to Campgaw to teach them skiing or snowboarding in a nonthreatening environment, while parents appreciate the chance to practice close to home.

The campsites at Campgaw generate similar reactions. Some wilderness buffs scoff at this urban forest, smack in the middle of Northern Jersey and less than 30 miles from Manhattan. The steady drone of traffic on Interstate 287 is always audible from the campground, reminding you that civilization is just past the nearest row of trees. But Campgaw's biggest handicap is also its major strength. A weekend camping expedition can begin as late as Saturday afternoon. The accessibility of Campgaw means families can show their kids how to sleep outdoors but can also break camp and drive home if the tots become grumpy and refuse to sleep.

Rustic sites line either side of a dead-end road. Some have parking but most are hike-in, although the hikes are little more than 40 feet. Visitors can leave their cars in one of three central parking areas. Five shelters dot the campground, and site borders are not clearly delineated. There are no privacy hedges and little understory, but sites are spacious and shaded. A few portable toilets line the road. Running water facilities are located in restrooms in the nearby cul-de-sac, near a grassy picnic area.

You must obtain a permit before setting up camp. These cannot be acquired on weekends or holidays, so plan ahead. Order them by mail or in person on week-

> *Campgaw's accessibility means a weekend camping expedition can start as late as Saturday afternoon.*

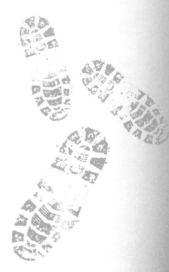

RATINGS

Beauty: ☆ ☆ ☆
Privacy: ☆ ☆
Spaciousness: ☆ ☆ ☆ ☆
Quiet: ☆ ☆
Security: ☆ ☆ ☆
Cleanliness: ☆ ☆

KEY INFORMATION

ADDRESS:	Campgaw Mountain Reservation 200 Campgaw Road Mahwah, NJ 07430
OPERATED BY:	Bergen County Department of Parks
INFORMATION:	(201) 327-3500
WEB SITE:	www.co.bergen.nj.us /parks
OPEN:	April 1–November 30
SITES:	18
EACH SITE HAS:	Picnic table, fire ring
ASSIGNMENT:	Choose from available sites
REGISTRATION:	In advance at Darlington County Parks office or by mail
FACILITIES:	Water, flush and vault toilets, showers
PARKING:	Lots near sites
FEE:	$10
ELEVATION:	450 feet
RESTRICTIONS:	**Pets:** On leash **Fires:** With fire permit only **Alcohol:** Prohibited **Vehicles:** No maximum **Other:** No swimming, wading, boating, or canoeing; no vehicles or bikes on trails

days from 9 a.m. to 4 p.m. at nearby Darlington County Park, 600 Darlington Road, Mahwah, NJ 07430, (201) 327-3500. Call ahead to discuss options and availability.

Campgaw Mountain is also home to a county-owned 28-station field archery range. Additionally, 18-hole Darlington County Golf Course is located across from the entrance on Campgaw Road. If you are visiting from out of town and wish to take a day trip into New York City, park your car 3 miles away at Ramsey train station. Catch the New Jersey Transit train to New York's Penn Station with a quick transfer at Secaucus Junction.

A small pond sits by the ski area, but swimming and boating are forbidden. Fishing is catch and release only. Additionally, hiking and bridle trails lace the 1,373-acre reservation. The concessionaire-operated Saddle Ridge Horseback Riding Center sits atop Campgaw Mountain and is accessible from nearby Franklin Lakes. Some of its offices and stables were originally built in the 1950s as part of the control area of Nike Battery NY-93/43, a program designed to launch guided surface-to-air missiles in the event of a Cold War Soviet attack. The launch site was located a mile north and has since been razed and turned into housing developments. New Jersey housed 14 Nike sites that were meant to protect New York and Philadelphia. The only one that was not destroyed is in Livingston, where the barracks and command center are preserved and open to the public at Riker Hill Park. The Nike missile program was named for the Greek goddess of victory, not for the popular running shoe.

The reservation features four easy and three moderate hiking trails. Only one, Old Cedar Trail, is more than a mile long. Combine this 2.1-mile trail with the Rocky Ridge Trail to form a longer 3-mile loop, which will take you to the top of the ski slope. Immediately after the trail crosses two stone walls near a ski slope building, you will see a white-blazed trail. Follow this a short way for panoramic views of the surrounding area. On clear days, you can see the Palisades and beyond to the Manhattan skyline. On humid summer days, don't expect to see much through the haze.

MAP

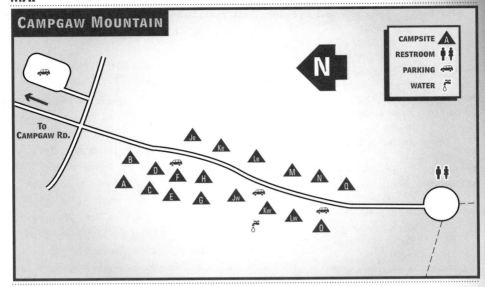

CAMPGAW MOUNTAIN

CAMPSITE	A
RESTROOM	👫
PARKING	🚗
WATER	🚰

N

To CAMPGAW RD.

Je, Ke, Le, B, D, F, H, A, C, E, G, Jw, M, N, Q, Kw, Lw, O

Access to Campgaw Mountain is easy for city and suburban dwellers. Aside from an RV park in Jersey City, this is the closest camping to New York City. As such, its mission is different than that of true wilderness campgrounds. In spite of this, Campgaw provides local families with great recreational activities and even a chance to view small wildlife (and possibly a few black bears) along with its access to the interstate.

GETTING THERE

From I-287, take Exit 66. Go 0.5 miles to US 202 South. Follow US 202 South for 1.7 miles to Darlington Avenue. Go left on Darlington Avenue for 0.3 miles. Turn right onto Campgaw Road. The park entrance is 1.1 miles on the right.

CAMP GLEN GRAY

> *A former Boy Scout camp, Glen Gray helped generations of boys learn to boat, fish, and respect nature on its 750 wooded acres.*

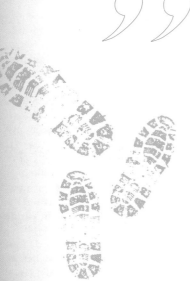

RUSTIC AND CONVENIENTLY LOCATED, Bergen County's newest campground is also its oldest. Camp Glen Gray was established in 1917 and developed over the next decade. For the next 85 years, it operated as a Boy Scouts of America camp. Generations of boys learned to boat, fish, respect nature, and cooperate on its 750 wooded acres.

Bergen County acquired the camp from the Boy Scouts in 2002, with help from the Trust for Public Land and a group of volunteers. The county provides mosquito control and snow removal, but for the most part, Camp Glen Gray is self-funded and managed by the Friends of Glen Gray Camp Operating Committee.

Ramapo Valley County Reservation is only 4.5 miles from Camp Glen Gray, and while both are wooded, primitive environments with great hiking trails, they serve different needs and different clienteles. Ramapo Valley is the top dog-walking and dog-camping destination in the region, and hundreds of people take their dogs through the park every day. Camp Glen Gray, however, does not allow visitors to bring dogs. Also, campsites at Ramapo are located near the entrance to the park, so every hiker passes by them. Wilderness camping at Camp Glen Gray is usually done in the North Quad, where campers who leave the trail are unlikely to see another human for the entire weekend. Ramapo Valley sites are well manicured, whereas Camp Glen Gray sites are more rugged.

All camping at Camp Glen Gray is hike-in, and the North Quad wilderness sites are ideal for solo campers or those hiking with a partner. Campers must leave their cars at the headquarters and hike to the backcountry along Old Guard Trail. It is also possible to hike in from other public lands via Cannonball Trail. All campers must check in and buy a permit at the headquarters. Wilderness camping at Glen Gray

RATINGS

Beauty: ✰ ✰ ✰
Privacy: ✰ ✰ ✰
Spaciousness: ✰ ✰
Quiet: ✰ ✰ ✰
Security: ✰ ✰ ✰
Cleanliness: ✰ ✰

offers no amenities, so campers must familiarize themselves with the basics of backcountry etiquette and bear behavior. Food should be carefully stored away from tents and campsites, preferably in bear-proof containers. Inquire at the office about the current bear population. All gear and garbage must be packed in and out.

Backcountry camping is possible at Camp Glen Gray, but the camp really shines in its offerings for families. The "Family Camp" weekends offer a taste of scouting without the Scouts. Children ages 6 through 12 and their families attend, staying in cabins, Glen Gray tents with cots, or their own tents. Meals are provided in the dining hall, and activities are offered throughout the weekend. Kids can swim, row boats on the small lake, fish, hike, or learn to make handicrafts. No-frills family weekends are also available, where families entertain themselves and cook over campfires.

Regular family camping is available on nonorganized (no workshops or classes) weekends. Campers stay in shady clearings that hold several tents. The entire clearing can be rented for $40 for a weekend, although most people rent cabins, so it's possible you'll have the clearing to yourself anyway. North Brook Campsite is one of the most popular clearings. It sits near the lake, close to amenities, and under hemlock trees on a bubbling stream. Swimming is prohibited unless a certified swim instructor is present. Rowboats are available for rent, but personal boats cannot be transported to the lake. Special arrangements with advance notification can be made for transportation for disabled campers.

Seven marked hiking trails wind through camp, in addition to many unmarked paths and trails that lead to other parts of the region. The white-blazed, 2-mile Millstone Trail is the most central. Easily accessed from the lake or office, it loops around camp, providing nice views from the top of Millstone Hill. The 4-mile Teepee Trail is popular for its view of New York City, some 45 miles away. Yellow Trail, Hoeferlin Memorial Trail, Schuber Trail, and Cannonball Trail cross the camp and are part of larger trail systems.

KEY INFORMATION

ADDRESS:	Camp Glen Gray 200 Midvale Mountain Road Mahwah, NJ 07430
OPERATED BY:	Friends of Glen Gray Camp Operating Committee
INFORMATION:	(201) 327-7234
WEB SITE:	www.glengray.org
OPEN:	Year-round weekends by permit; weekdays by special reservation
SITES:	150, plus unlimited wilderness sites
EACH SITE HAS:	No amenities in wilderness sites; picnic table, fire ring, some platforms
ASSIGNMENT:	In advance
REGISTRATION:	In advance, by phone or Web site
FACILITIES:	Latrines, showers, water (limited in winter)
PARKING:	Central lot, hike-in
FEE:	$3 per person for weekend; $40 for entire clearing per weekend
ELEVATION:	635 feet
RESTRICTIONS:	Pets: Prohibited Fires: By permit only Alcohol: Prohibited Vehicles: At parking area Other: Use dumpster near office; licensed fishing only; no hunting; swimming only with certified lifeguard; no bikes

MAP

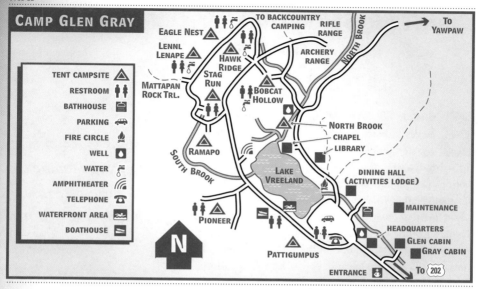

CAMP GLEN GRAY

Legend:
- TENT CAMPSITE
- RESTROOM
- BATHHOUSE
- PARKING
- FIRE CIRCLE
- WELL
- WATER
- AMPHITHEATER
- TELEPHONE
- WATERFRONT AREA
- BOATHOUSE

Map labels:
EAGLE NEST
LENNI LENAPE
MATTAPAN ROCK TRL.
STAG RUN
HAWK RIDGE
BOBCAT HOLLOW
TO BACKCOUNTRY CAMPING
RIFLE RANGE
ARCHERY RANGE
NORTH BROOK
To YAWPAW
RAMAPO
SOUTH BROOK
LAKE VREELAND
NORTH BROOK CHAPEL
LIBRARY
DINING HALL (ACTIVITIES LODGE)
MAINTENANCE
PIONEER
PATTIGUMPUS
HEADQUARTERS
GLEN CABIN
GRAY CABIN
ENTRANCE
To 202
N

GETTING THERE

From I-287, take Exit 58. Turn onto US 202 North. Drive 1.9 miles to Glen Gray Road. Turn left and go over the steel bridge. Turn right onto Midvale Mountain Road. Continue 0.6 mile to the camp entrance.

Camp Glen Gray rents out its facilities to groups year-round. It has almost unlimited space for medium-sized groups but limited parking and is at the end of a private road. Campers are encouraged to stay at camp all weekend rather than constantly drive in and out. Bear in mind that the facilities are not new. Campers seeking a rustic outdoors experience will be pleased here, but those who require modern plumbing and drive-in sites will be better served setting up tents at nearby Campgaw Mountain Reservation.

RAMAPO VALLEY COUNTY RESERVATION

BERGEN COUNTY, with 884,000 people, has the largest human population of any of New Jersey's counties. Its canine population cannot be far behind, and you will see a large cross-section of both as people and dogs enjoy the trails and ponds of Ramapo Valley County Reservation.

Nine tent campsites surround 22-acre Scarlet Oak Pond, while the remaining single tent site is just across the footbridge on the banks of the Ramapo River. All sites are hike-in only because the park's entire 3,313 acres are closed to vehicles. The hike from the parking area to Scarlet Oak Pond is a short 200 yards. The restrooms, with sinks and flushing toilets, are located near the parking area. There are no showers.

All sites are adjacent to trails traveled by day hikers, but sites 7 through 10 are isolated from the others, providing slightly more privacy. Ramapo Valley County Reservation closes a half hour after sunset, and the crowds disperse, leaving behind a bucolic scene where campers sleep on spacious grassy areas under the stars, the silence broken only by the sound of the gurgling river.

Early morning brings back the urban refugees. Join the fisherfolk by pulling on rubber waders and fly-fishing or casting for trout in the seasonally stocked Scarlet Oak Pond or Ramapo River. Catfish, panfish, perch, and bass are also present. Signs indicate when trout stocking occurs and whether it is taking place in the pond, river, or both. New Jersey fishing licenses are required for those over age 16.

Fifteen miles of moderately difficult trails wind through this hilly former farmland. Free maps with GPS coordinates are available at a kiosk in the parking lot. The steep green-on-white-blazed Halifax Trail, which begins on the west side of Scarlet Oak Pond, is recommended for its access to Hawk Rock, a ledge fea-

> *Signs warn of bears, but you're more likely to encounter throngs of happy mutts straining at their leashes.*

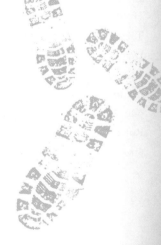

RATINGS

Beauty: ☆ ☆ ☆
Privacy: ☆
Spaciousness: ☆ ☆ ☆ ☆
Quiet: ☆ ☆
Security: ☆ ☆
Cleanliness: ☆ ☆ ☆

ADDRESS:	Ramapo Valley County Reservation 584 Ramapo Valley Road Mahwah, NJ 07430
OPERATED BY:	Bergen County Department of Parks
INFORMATION:	(201) 327-3500
WEB SITE:	www.co.bergen.nj.us /parks
OPEN:	April 1–November 30
SITES:	10
EACH SITE HAS:	Picnic table, fire ring
ASSIGNMENT:	Choose from available sites
REGISTRATION:	In advance at Darlington County Parks office or by mail
FACILITIES:	Water, flush toilets
PARKING:	Central lot, hike-in
FEE:	$10 for up to 6 people
ELEVATION:	250 feet
RESTRICTIONS:	**Pets:** Dogs must be on leash shorter than 6 feet **Fires:** By permit only **Alcohol:** Prohibited **Vehicles:** At parking area **Other:** Carry out all trash (dumpster in parking lot); licensed fishing only; no hunting; no swimming; no bikes on trails; no boating

turing outstanding views of Bergen County and Manhattan. Go early on humid summer days to avoid the haze that can descend over New York City.

A second lookout with a view of Campgaw Mountain and Manhattan is on the blue-blazed Ridge Trail. From the intersection of Silver Macmillan Trail and Blue Ridge Trail, walk 0.3 mile along Ridge Trail to find the lookout turnoff.

Another popular route is the yellow-blazed Waterfall Trail. The falls have been described as both "incredible" and "barely visible" depending on recent rains. The more popular trails are less likely to be inhabited by wildlife, but hiking farther out may produce sightings of pheasant and deer. Snakes are common at Ramapo Valley, particularly near the dam. Be considerate and avoid them if possible.

Three trails—Cannonball, Hoeferlin, and Crossover—are maintained by volunteers from the NY/NJ Trail Conference. These continue through Ringwood State Park and the Ramapo Mountains.

Camping and fires are allowed by permit only, and late arrivals without permits are forbidden to camp. Vehicles left in the parking area without permits may be towed. All campers are required to pack out their garbage. New Jersey has an overpopulation of black bears, so be careful not to leave food or waste products. Bicycles are not allowed on the trails, so leave bikes behind on the parking lot bike rack.

Permits are available in person or by mail on weekdays from 9 a.m. to 4 p.m. at nearby Darlington County Park, 600 Darlington Road, Mahwah, NJ 07430. The office is closed on holidays. If you plan on arriving after office hours or on a weekend, apply for a permit in advance by mail or phone. Plan ahead for busy summer weekends; sites are limited. Ramapo Valley sites are in demand because state campgrounds in New Jersey do not allow dogs to stay overnight.

As you leave your site for your day's activities, keep in mind that hundreds of people may pass your tent during the day. Tent burglary is not a problem at Ramapo Valley County Reservation, and enough people are around to discourage would-be thieves, but consider locking valuables in the car as a preventive measure.

MAP

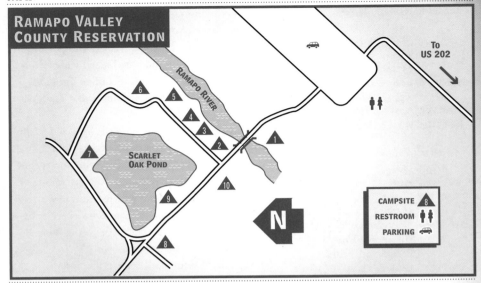

RAMAPO VALLEY
COUNTY RESERVATION

RAMAPO RIVER

To
US 202

6
5
4
3
2
1

7

SCARLET
OAK POND

10

9

N

8

CAMPSITE   8
RESTROOM   👫
PARKING   🚗

The camping area is only occasionally patrolled by the Bergen County Park Security Department.

Only 35 miles from Manhattan, Ramapo Valley County Reservation caters to thousands as a wilderness area adjacent to an urban environment. Its hiking trails are populated by urban refugees anxious for a green hike. Signs warn of bears, but you're more likely to encounter throngs of happy mutts straining at their leashes.

GETTING THERE

From I-287, take Exit 66.
Turn onto US 202 South.
Drive 1.8 miles to the park
entrance on the right.

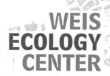

WEIS ECOLOGY CENTER

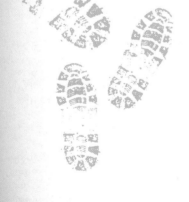

> *Weis Ecology Center campground caters to tenters only, especially those truly wishing to get back to nature.*

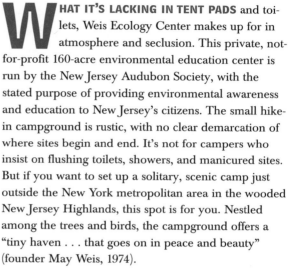

WHAT IT'S LACKING IN TENT PADS and toilets, Weis Ecology Center makes up for in atmosphere and seclusion. This private, not-for-profit 160-acre environmental education center is run by the New Jersey Audubon Society, with the stated purpose of providing environmental awareness and education to New Jersey's citizens. The small hike-in campground is rustic, with no clear demarcation of where sites begin and end. It's not for campers who insist on flushing toilets, showers, and manicured sites. But if you want to set up a solitary, scenic camp just outside the New York metropolitan area in the wooded New Jersey Highlands, this spot is for you. Nestled among the trees and birds, the campground offers a "tiny haven . . . that goes on in peace and beauty" (founder May Weis, 1974).

Facilities are minimal and primitive at the campground. You must bring your own water and remove your trash. Campers may use the flushing toilets and showers in the basement of the Reception Center during the day, but after 4:30 p.m. the buildings are locked and campers have access only to latrines at the entrance to the camping area. All sites are hike-in only. Cars can be left by permit only at a central lot along a small creek. The easy hike in is less than a half mile.

Campsites are open year-round, and primitive cabins and rooms are available for rent April through October. Cabins are available for seasonal rentals. Weis Ecology Center, including overnight options, is only open Wednesday through Sunday, although the grounds are open daily. Advance reservations are required for camping as well as for cabin rental. Call ahead to confirm your spot—and to ensure you will not be camping in the middle of a Scout or school group environmental education weekend.

Weis Ecology Center is adjacent to the 4,365-acre

RATINGS

Beauty: ☆ ☆ ☆ ☆
Site privacy: ☆ ☆ ☆ ☆
Spaciousness: ☆ ☆ ☆ ☆
Quiet: ☆ ☆ ☆ ☆
Security: ☆ ☆
Cleanliness: ☆ ☆

Norvin Green State Forest, an undeveloped wilderness sanctuary that offers hiking along old logging roads and new trails built by volunteers. The state forest has no parking lots of its own, so leave your car in the lot at Weis or park along Burnt Meadow Road or Glen Wild Road. Trails stretch through rugged terrain. Some are challenging, with hills ranging from 400 to 1,300 feet, so be prepared.

The blue-blazed Hewitt Butler Trail is popular for its views of 25-foot-high Chikahoki Falls and 15-foot-high Otter Hole. Many seasonal waterfalls dot the area, so be sure to pick up a map at Weis Ecology Center before wandering into the woods. The red-blazed Wyanokie Circular Trail, which begins on Snake Den Road, climbs 500 feet to Wyanokie High Point. This area features views of the Wanaque Reservoir and surrounding mountains. On clear days, the New York City skyline is visible, some 40 miles away.

Sections of Wyanokie Circular Trail, the Hewitt-Butler Trails, and Wyanokie Crest Trail are part of the 150-mile-long Highlands Trail, a cooperative venture between the New York–New Jersey Trail Conference and various conservation groups. The Highlands Trail enters the Newark Watershed immediately south of the area. A permit is required to hike there.

The short hike to Blue Mine Falls is an easy outing, but if you wind around the yellow and red trails, you will see some old mines. Iron ore was discovered in the area in 1765, and mines were worked until the late 1800s. The last mine was shut down in 1905, and the first trail opened eight years later. Dr. Will S. Monroe, a professor from Montclair, planned most of the trails in the Wyanokie area. Weis Ecology Center was established in 1974 by Walter and May Weis, and about 12,000 people visit it every year.

In addition to hiking and overnight facilities, Weis Ecology Center has a butterfly and songbird meadow, an aviary that houses permanently injured birds of prey, a stream-fed swimming pool, and a variety of day and outreach programs.

Programs include interpretive hikes, maple sugaring lectures, shelter building, and wildlife ecology. Lessons are given on compass reading and orienteer-

KEY INFORMATION

ADDRESS:	Weis Ecology Center 150 Snake Den Road Ringwood, NJ 07456
OPERATED BY:	New Jersey Audubon Society
INFORMATION:	(973) 835-2160
WEB SITE:	www.njaudubon.org
OPEN:	Year-round Wednesday–Sunday; closed holiday Mondays; gates locked November 1–April 1; campers must walk in
SITES:	10
EACH SITE HAS:	Picnic table, fire ring
ASSIGNMENT:	Reservations required
REGISTRATION:	Register at office before 4 p.m.; advance reservations and signature for fire permit required
FACILITIES:	Latrines, toilets, showers, potable water at reception center (closes at 4:30 p.m.)
PARKING:	At designated lot; short hike to sites
FEE:	$3.50 per person
ELEVATION:	550 feet
RESTRICTIONS:	**Pets:** Prohibited **Fires:** Allowed by permit only in fire rings **Alcohol:** Prohibited **Vehicles:** Prohibited **Other:** Campers may use dead materials found on forest floor for fires; quiet hours begin at 10 p.m.; no radios or loud noise

MAP

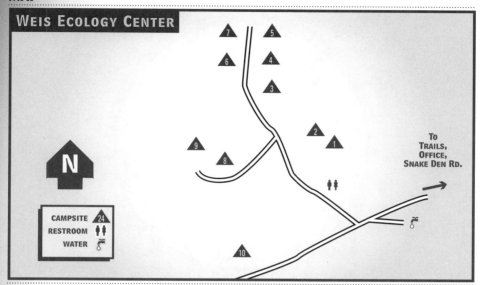

WEIS ECOLOGY CENTER

N

To TRAILS, OFFICE, SNAKE DEN RD.

CAMPSITE 24
RESTROOM
WATER

GETTING THERE

From I-287, take Exit 55. Turn right at the end of the ramp onto Ringwood Avenue (County Road 511 North). Ringwood Avenue veers left at a T-intersection. Continue for 4 miles. Turn left onto Westbrook Road. Bear left at the fork. Take the second left onto Snake Den Road. Bear left at the fork again and drive 0.3 miles to Weis Ecology Center.

ing. Birds, insects, and trees are examined, and occasionally guided hikes into an abandoned iron mine are offered. Live animal programs include site visits to schools in which snakes, birds, or reptiles might be part of the lesson program.

The unpolished sites and natural trails of Weis hold limited appeal for many. But those seeking a secluded, unaffected environment and a little ecological education should pay a visit to this rural oasis in an urban environment.

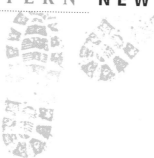

WESTERN NEW JERSEY

CAMP TAYLOR

SET ON A REMOTE HILLSIDE on the ridge of the Kittatinny Mountains, this private campground offers an unusual and appealing mix of attractions. Camp Taylor's wooded hillside tenting area, with primitive sites that are both spacious and shaded, is only part of its appeal. The remote location is another draw; the 350-acre camp is adjacent to 70,000-acre Delaware Water Gap National Recreation Area, which is quite large for a backyard. Camp Taylor offers organized activities for both kids and adults and a miniature golf course, a swimming area, and a game room. But what truly distinguishes Camp Taylor from the pack is its own pack; it has an on-site wolf preserve.

Lakota Wolf Preserve features four wildlife pens dispersed over ten acres. Three of the football field–sized pens are for adult timber, tundra, and arctic wolves. The fourth pen houses foxes, bobcats, and wolf pups. The animals have all been raised in captivity and are habituated to humans, so they do not hide when visitors stop by. Wolf watches (which include feedings) happen twice daily, although there is no guarantee you will see the wolves playing and wandering around. They do tend to come out at feeding times though, so you'll have an excellent chance of seeing them eat. Wolf watches and feedings happen at 10:30 a.m. year-round, while the afternoon watch occurs at 4 p.m. in summer and 3 p.m. during the rest of the year. Through lectures, visitors also learn about the social structure of wolf packs, the wolves' daily lives, and their eating habits. Reservations are necessary for weekday wolf watches, but no appointments are necessary on weekends. Pets are prohibited from going on wolf watches. Camp management recommends boarding your animal at Vom Rohaus Kennels on Route 94 in Hainesburg during your wolf watch. Noncampers can also visit and view the wolves on wolf-watch walks.

> *What distinguishes Camp Taylor from th pack is its own pack; it has an on-site wolf preserve.*

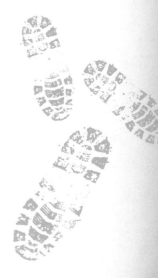

RATINGS

Beauty: ✿ ✿ ✿
Privacy: ✿ ✿
Spaciousness: ✿ ✿ ✿
Quiet: ✿ ✿ ✿
Security: ✿ ✿ ✿ ✿
Cleanliness: ✿ ✿ ✿

ADDRESS: Camp Taylor Campground
85 Mount Pleasant Road
Columbia, NJ 07832

OPERATED BY: Private

INFORMATION: (908) 496-4333

WEB SITE: www.camptaylor.com

OPEN: Mid-April–October, off-season by reservation

SITES: 24

EACH SITE HAS: Picnic table, fire ring

ASSIGNMENT: Choose from available sites

REGISTRATION: On arrival or by reservation (2-day minimum for weekend reservations)

FACILITIES: Water, flush toilets, showers

PARKING: At site or in lot

FEE: 2 people, $20; additional adult, $10; children ages 2–11, $2.50; children ages 12–15, $5

ELEVATION: 800 feet

RESTRICTIONS: **Pets:** On leash only; one per site; cannot go near wolves
Fires: In fire rings only
Alcohol: At site
Vehicles: Up to 38 feet
Other: Quiet hours 11 p.m.–9 a.m.; check-in 4 p.m. or later

Wolf walks involve a 0.5-mile hike through the forest. Transportation is available if visitors cannot walk that distance; call the campground for details. Photographers should note that a chain-link fence sits between wolves and visitors. Professional photographers can schedule private photo sessions for a fee.

The wolves eat between 30,000 and 40,000 pounds of meat a year. They get a lot of local roadkill—New Jersey has an abundance of deer that wander onto roadways. But the bulk of their food comes from Space Farms Zoo on Route 519 in Sussex County. The private zoo, originally a general store, began as a roadside attraction in 1927. Goliath, a 12-foot-tall Alaskan brown bear and its star attraction for many years, is now stuffed and on display in the gift shop.

Camp Taylor gets busy on summer weekends, and they require a two-night minimum for reservations, which are highly recommended. Campsites are open mid-April through October, but year-round camping is possible by advance reservation. Three vault toilets service the tent camping area, and flush toilets and showers are a long hike away at the office. Some tent sites provide more understory and privacy than others, so arrive early and choose carefully. All sites feature shade. The usual warnings about camping in bear country apply: use bear-proof containers and never take food into or near your tent. See the Introduction for more information on how to camp safely in bear country. Camp Taylor provides trash containers at each site, as well as centrally located recycling barrels.

Fishing is prohibited at the campground, but swimming is allowed in the two-acre lake. Nonswimmers must stay in the immediate beach area and must be accompanied by an adult swimmer at all times. Paddleboats and kayaks are available for rent. Anglers enjoy nearby Delaware and Paulinskill rivers.

Campers who tire of the game room, volleyball court, and organized activities can take to the trails. Mountain Trail leaves Camp Taylor property behind the farthest wildlife pen and meets up with a fire road right inside public lands. Hike to the left for 2.2 miles to reach the Delaware Water Gap National Recreation Area and the trail up Mount Tammany. Take a right

MAP

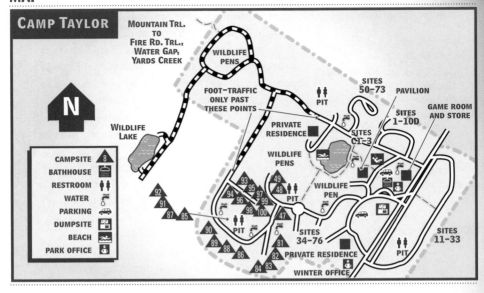

and the same length hike will take you to Yards Creek, where walking trails surround a power facility. You can also access the famed Appalachian Trail from Yards Creek.

Even without the wolf preserve, Camp Taylor stands on its own as a decent campground. Sites are wooded, and campers will find plenty of activities to keep both children and adults occupied. But the wolf preserve elevates this campground from a nicely wooded private area to an utterly unique experience.

GETTING THERE

From I-80, take Exit 4, then take NJ 94 north for 3.5 miles. Turn left onto Benton Road. Make a right at Frog Pond Road. Go left onto Wishing Well. Turn left at the end of the road. Campground entrance is on the right.

DELAWARE WATER GAP NATIONAL RECREATION AREA (CANOE-IN)

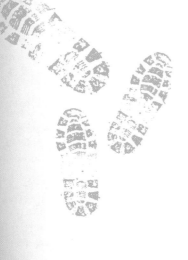

> *More than 100 free canoe-in campsites dot the Delaware River.*

THE SHALLOW, GENTLE DELAWARE RIVER hardly seems powerful enough to wash away a sandbar, much less a chunk of mountain. But centuries ago, this unassuming body of water carved an 1,100-foot-deep, 3-mile-long gorge out of the solid rock of the Kittatinny Ridge.

Canoeists have used this part of the Delaware for travel since the days of the Lenape Native Americans, but today's boaters are more interested in scenery and recreation than in transportation. Mount Tammany rises above the river on the Jersey side, and Mount Minis overshadows it on the Pennsylvania side. The Delaware Water Gap National Recreation Area stretches north from the gap for 40 miles, encompassing 70,000 acres of land along both sides of the river.

The National Park Service administers the recreation area and runs no developed campgrounds within its boundaries. Those with cars or trailers must rely upon the sites at Worthington State Forest or nearby private campgrounds. But for campers willing to rough it on the water, leaving cars, RVs, and heaviest amenities at home, there are plenty of campsites in the Delaware Water Gap.

More than 100 canoe-in primitive campsites dot the Delaware between Kittatinny Point at the Gap and Mashipacong Island at the northern end of the park. Many sites are inaccessible without a boat. And even if you have a boat, campers cannot just canoe in, camp, and then canoe back to their cars at the nearest boat ramp. Nor is it acceptable for campers to leave their cars by the side of the road and hike to a campsite. The Delaware Water Gap National Recreation Area canoe-in sites are meant for boaters, but not just any boaters. Canoeists must be on what the park service terms "bona fide overnight trips," meaning trips long enough to merit an overnight stop.

RATINGS

Beauty: ✿ ✿ ✿ ✿
Privacy: ✿ ✿ ✿
Spaciousness: ✿ ✿
Quiet: ✿ ✿ ✿
Security: ✿ ✿
Cleanliness: ✿ ✿

One-night trips that are defined as "bona fide" are trips that go from either Milford Beach to Eshback (or farther); Dingmans Ferry or Eshback to Smithfield Beach (or farther); Bushkill to Kittatinny Point (or farther). Two-night trips that merit camping are from Milford Beach to Smithfield Beach (or farther) and Dingmans Ferry to Kittatinny Point (or farther). The only trip requiring three nights of camping begins at the northernmost access point at Milford Beach and goes the length of the park to Kittatinny Point. All camping is limited to one night per site.

Some sites are on islands, while others are located on the banks on either the New Jersey or the Pennsylvania sides of the river. Several are isolated individual sites, others are clustered together. Some have vault toilets, others have no facilities at all, which means latrines must be dug. Drinking water is not available at most sites, and river water is not recommended for drinking; bring your own. Carry out all garbage. Remember, bears live in the area, so use bear-proof containers and never take food into or near your tent.

Alcohol is prohibited while paddling, at all times in Worthington State Forest, and between Depew Island and Dupue Island on the Pennsylvania side of the park. Canoeists should remember that alcohol and canoeing can be a deadly combination. Rangers can remove you from the river if you appear intoxicated.

The National Park Service does not offer shuttles or canoe rentals, but more than 20 liveries are licensed to rent gear and transport boaters between access points. Children under 12 years old are required to wear life jackets, and people of all ages are encouraged to wear them. The Delaware River has no difficult rapids, and access points appear every 8 to 10 miles. Visit during a shoulder season or midweek if you can, as the river gets crowded on summer weekends.

As a recreation area, the park is surprisingly undeveloped. It has been public property since 1965, when the Delaware Water Gap National Recreation Area was established, but it was not instantly developed into public parkland. For ten years, the government and environmental groups wrestled over a plan to dam the river, flooding nearby towns and villages to build the

KEY INFORMATION

ADDRESS: Delaware Water Gap National Recreation Area Headquarters River Road off Route 209 Bushkill, PA 18324

OPERATED BY: National Park Service

INFORMATION: (570) 588-2452

WEB SITE: www.nps.gov/dewa

OPEN: Year-round

SITES: 100

EACH SITE HAS: Some with fire ring, some with vault toilet

ASSIGNMENT: First come, first served

REGISTRATION: None required

FEE: Free camping; $5 vehicle fee at Milford Beach, Smithfield Beach, Bushkill Dingmans Ferry

ELEVATION: 340 feet

RESTRICTIONS: Pets: On short leash Fires: In fire rings only; okay to collect downed wood Alcohol: Prohibited while boating; prohibited from Depew Island to Dupue Island Vehicles: None Other: 1-night stay a part of multiday river trip only; camp only at designated sites; carry out all trash; no cutting of live trees; wash away from water sources; bury pet and human waste 6 inches underground and at least 300 feet from water; no excessive noise; quiet hours 10 p.m.–6 a.m.

MAP

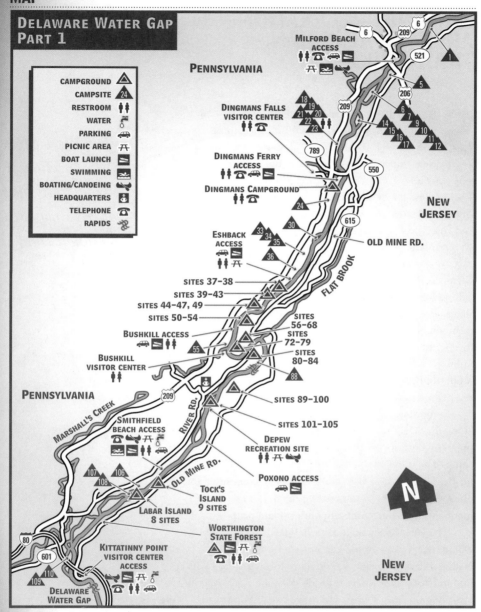

DELAWARE WATER GAP PART 1

Legend

- CAMPGROUND
- CAMPSITE
- RESTROOM
- WATER
- PARKING
- PICNIC AREA
- BOAT LAUNCH
- SWIMMING
- BOATING/CANOEING
- HEADQUARTERS
- TELEPHONE
- RAPIDS

PENNSYLVANIA

MILFORD BEACH ACCESS

DINGMANS FALLS VISITOR CENTER

DINGMANS FERRY ACCESS

DINGMANS CAMPGROUND

ESHBACK ACCESS

OLD MINE RD.

NEW JERSEY

FLAT BROOK

SITES 37–38
SITES 39–43
SITES 44–47, 49
SITES 50–54

SITES 56–68
SITES 72–79

BUSHKILL ACCESS

SITES 80–84

BUSHKILL VISITOR CENTER

PENNSYLVANIA

MARSHALL'S CREEK

SITES 89–100

SITES 101–105

SMITHFIELD BEACH ACCESS

DEPEW RECREATION SITE

POXONO ACCESS

TOCK'S ISLAND 9 SITES

LABAR ISLAND 8 SITES

WORTHINGTON STATE FOREST

KITTATINNY POINT VISITOR CENTER ACCESS

DELAWARE WATER GAP

NEW JERSEY

OLD MINE RD.

RIVER RD.

GETTING THERE

From I-80 at the Delaware Water Gap, access to boat launches are from points north along Old Mine Rd. (NJ side) and US 209 (PA side).

Tocks Island Dam. Thousands of residents were displaced, and many of their homes destroyed. The plan fell apart in 1975 and was officially deauthorized in 1992. The property remained public. Many plans for the recreation area are just being initiated today. Take advantage of the lazy rivers and isolated campsites while they last.

DELAWARE WATER GAP NATIONAL RECREATION AREA/APPALACHIAN TRAIL (HIKE-IN)

SETTING UP CAMP in the Delaware Water Gap along the Appalachian Trail isn't something you do on a whim. You can't park your car nearby, lug your gear up a hill, drag along the cooler, and erect a tent. No, camping along the Appalachian Trail in New Jersey's heavily used Delaware Water Gap National Recreation Area is limited to designated areas and reserved exclusively for hikers on trips that require an overnight stop.

As most hikers know, the Appalachian National Scenic Trail (or A.T.) traverses mountain ridges and valleys for 2,100 miles as it winds its way across 14 states. The Garden State, although this term seems a misnomer on the craggy Kittatinny Range, is crossed by 73.6 of those miles. The Delaware Water Gap's 27.3 miles get a lot of use, particularly on weekends when urban refugees leave New York City and Northern Jersey behind and take to the remote trails.

Some states allow dispersed backcountry camping along the A.T. New Jersey is one of three states that precisely designates where hikers can and cannot camp. The other two states are New York and Connecticut, both heavy-use states. Hikers are reminded to obey these rules both to preserve the natural environment and to avoid stumbling onto private property.

The New Jersey State Park Service is picky about where hikers can camp while in state forests, but the National Park Service is a little more forgiving. You will find only one spot where trailside camping is allowed in Worthington State Forest, and Stokes State Forest welcomes campers with a sign forbidding them to camp for the next 4 miles. In between state property is federal land, and hikers are allowed to set up tents within 100 feet of the trail, but there are rules to follow.

Aside from the rule that hikers must be on trips requiring an overnight stop, hikers must not camp

> *Free primitive campin[g]*
> *along this section of th[e]*
> *A.T. is reserved for hi[k]-*
> *ers on trips requiring*
> *an overnight stop.*

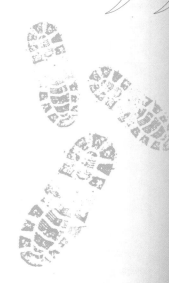

RATINGS

Beauty: ✿ ✿ ✿ ✿ ✿
Privacy: ✿ ✿ ✿
Spaciousness: ✿ ✿ ✿
Quiet: ✿ ✿ ✿ ✿ ✿
Security: ✿ ✿
Cleanliness: ✿ ✿ ✿

KEY INFORMATION

ADDRESS: Delaware Water Gap
National Recreation
Area Headquarters
River Road off
US 209
Bushkill, PA 18324

OPERATED BY: National Park
Service

INFORMATION: (570) 588-2452

WEB SITE: www.nps.gov/dewa

OPEN: Year-round

SITES: Wilderness camping

EACH SITE HAS: No amenities

ASSIGNMENT: Choose available
spot within
designated area

REGISTRATION: Not required

FACILITIES: None

PARKING: At designated lots;
hike-in to sites

FEE: Free

ELEVATION: Varies

RESTRICTIONS: Pets: On leash
Fires: Prohibited
Alcohol: Prohibited
Vehicles: Prohibited
Other: 1-night limit
per campsite; no
camping within 200
feet of other
campers; carry out
all trash; camping
restricted to those
hiking 2 or more
days; camp within
100 feet of trail

within 100 feet of a water source or within 200 feet of another party. Camping is prohibited within a half mile of a roadway and from a half mile south of Blue Mountain Lake to 1 mile north of Crater Lake. Hikers may not start ground fires but can use camp stoves.

The 4 miles from Dunnfield Trailhead to Sunfish Pond are used heavily by day hikers. Nevertheless, enough thru-hikers stop at the single campsite within the Worthington State Forest section that the site is often crowded. But it is not used by many who begin their hikes at the Dunnfield parking area. Sites farther on, past the Worthington boundary and inside federal lands, are more promising and more spread out. Some sites are utilitarian, best for the exhausted, while others are scenic and private, requiring short side hikes.

Remember, bears live in the area, so use bear-proof containers and never take food into or near your tent. See the Introduction for more information on how to camp safely in bear country.

Snakes inhabit the woods but are shy and seldom encountered by people. Avoid them if you see them. Few snakebites have been reported along the Appalachian Trail. Hikers should take precautions against ticks, as many of them carry Lyme Disease. Some mosquitoes transmit West Nile Virus. Wear insecticide and sleeves if possible.

National Park Service regulations state that hikers must carry enough water for their entire hike within the Delaware Water Gap. You will find water along the trail, but it is unreliable and often contaminated. With advance research, campers can learn of water sources, but you must chemically treat the water or boil it for five minutes prior to ingestion. All trash must be carried out. Campers are reminded that these campsites are for overnight hikers, which means you must familiarize yourself with not only the rules of the A.T. but also with the basics of overnight hikes. Read some books on A.T. hiking and talk to staff at the New York–New Jersey Trail Conference (www.nynjtc.com) before setting out for your first overnight hike.

The Delaware Water Gap Recreation Area covers 68,000 acres on both the New Jersey and Pennsylvania sides of the Delaware River. Views are most

MAP

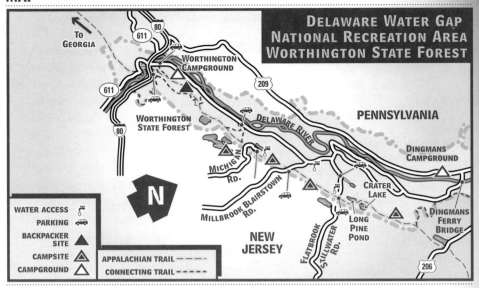

**DELAWARE WATER GAP
NATIONAL RECREATION AREA
WORTHINGTON STATE FOREST**

To GEORGIA

80
611

209

611

80

WORTHINGTON
CAMPGROUND

WORTHINGTON
STATE FOREST

DELAWARE RIVER

PENNSYLVANIA

DINGMANS
CAMPGROUND

MICHIGAN RD.

MILLBROOK BLAIRSTOWN RD.

CRATER
LAKE

N

NEW
JERSEY

LONG
PINE
POND

DINGMANS
FERRY
BRIDGE

FLATBROOK STILLWATER RD.

206

WATER ACCESS
PARKING
BACKPACKER
SITE
CAMPSITE
CAMPGROUND

APPALACHIAN TRAIL — — ·
CONNECTING TRAIL - - - - -

spectacular either from the river looking up or from scenic overlooks along the Kittatinny Ridge. Once hikers leave federal property and enter state property in Stokes State Forest and High Point State Park, they must camp in shelters. But along the A.T. in New Jersey, hikers will find some of the nicest primitive campsites in the state.

GETTING THERE

From I-80 heading west toward the NJ–PA border, take Exit 1 and follow signs to the Ranger Station, then signs to Dunnfield parking area. Or exit to the parking area—rest stop immediately after mile marker 1. Parking at the northern end is at Culvers Gap on US 206.

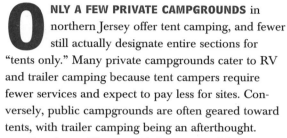

Branchville

HARMONY RIDGE CAMPGROUND

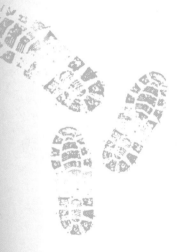

> *Harmony Ridge is perfect for families who want to explore nearby natural areas while still keeping Fido in tow.*

ONLY A FEW PRIVATE CAMPGROUNDS in northern Jersey offer tent camping, and fewer still actually designate entire sections for "tents only." Many private campgrounds cater to RV and trailer camping because tent campers require fewer services and expect to pay less for sites. Conversely, public campgrounds are often geared toward tents, with trailer camping being an afterthought.

Family-run Harmony Ridge is one of those rare private campgrounds that encourages tent camping. Section O and its 28 tent sites are set off by themselves in a shaded, level grove. The small dirt road discourages RV owners. RV sites are spacious and not crammed together as they are at many private campgrounds. The entire campground has been carefully landscaped and is impeccably maintained.

The three rustic campgrounds of Stokes State Forest are nearby, and some may wonder what the benefit is of staying in a pricier private site when $15 tent sites are right over the ridge past the Appalachian Trail (A.T). Camping can be different things to different people. For some, the ideal campsite is a small wooded clearing with a pit toilet and no neighbors in site. For others, particularly those with families, the best campsites come with organized activities and amenities.

Harmony Ridge, with its game room, whirlpool, and shady tent sites, provides the best mixture for those families needing some modern conveniences along with their forests and hiking trails. But modern amenities are not the only appeal at Harmony Ridge. Dogs, prohibited in New Jersey state campgrounds, are allowed to stay at Harmony Ridge campsites.

Head up to Section H to find the hiking trail. From the last RV site, it's less than a mile's walk to the A.T. and the Normanook (Culver) fire tower. A favorite walk of many local hikers is the trail section

RATINGS

Beauty: ☆ ☆ ☆
Privacy: ☆ ☆
Spaciousness: ☆ ☆ ☆
Quiet: ☆ ☆
Security: ☆ ☆ ☆ ☆
Cleanliness: ☆ ☆ ☆ ☆

that goes from the fire tower to Sunrise Mountain. If
the fire tower is unattended, you may be able to climb
up for a view. Then walk about 3.5 miles north to
1,653 feet at Sunrise Mountain. Relax at the summit in
the pavilion built in the 1930s by the Civilian Conservation Corps (CCC) and take in the panorama of surrounding Sussex County. Hike early if recent days
have been hazy. Several of the trails nearby continue
into Stokes State Forest, while the A.T. goes north from
Stokes through High Point State Park, eventually
reaching Maine.

After breaking in your hiking shoes, you can relax
back at Harmony Ridge's pool or beach. Fish (catch
and release) for largemouth bass, catfish, or bluegill in
one of the three stocked lakes. Play basketball, shuffleboard, boccie, horseshoes, miniature golf, or volleyball
(on sand brought north from Cape May). Or simply sit
at a campfire and do nothing.

Ed and Doris Ann Risdon opened Harmony
Ridge with just ten campsites in 1966. Today there are
20 times more sites on the 160-acre property, as well as
several more Risdons. The family still manages and
oversees the operation, which includes organized activities in addition to recreational facilities. Harmony
Ridge offers RV and cabin rentals in addition to tent
and trailer camping.

Campers receive an informational booklet at
check-in, which includes campground policies, a guide
to local restaurants and attractions, activity descrip-
tions, and a guide to local wildlife. Hand-drawn rac-
coons, beavers, deer, turkeys, birds, and foxes are
some of the animals shown. Campers can check off the
wildlife they see as they hike the nearby trails.

Another nearby private tent camping option is
Beaver Hill Campground, 10 miles to the southeast.
Primarily an RV park, Beaver Hill offers 12 tent-only
sites on a shaded hill that overlooks the bathhouse.
Recreational facilities are similar to Harmony Ridge's,
but the campground is smaller and does not have
backyard access to the Appalachian Trail.

For families (especially those with dogs) wishing to
experience outdoor living, there are times when a
secluded campsite on New Jersey public property is

KEY INFORMATION

ADDRESS:	Harmony Ridge Campground 23 Risdon Drive Branchville, NJ 07826
OPERATED BY:	State Park Service
INFORMATION:	(973) 948-4941
WEB SITE:	www.harmony ridge.com
OPEN:	Year-round
SITES:	28 tent sites (228 total sites)
EACH SITE HAS:	Picnic table, fire ring
ASSIGNMENT:	Choose from available sites
REGISTRATION:	On arrival or by reservation
FACILITIES:	Water, flush toilets, showers, pay phone, laundry
PARKING:	At site
FEE:	Adult, $15; child, $5
ELEVATION:	900 feet
RESTRICTIONS:	Pets: On leash; not allowed in rental trailers or cabins Fires: In fire rings only Alcohol: At site Vehicles: Up to 40 feet Other: 2-night minimum

MAP

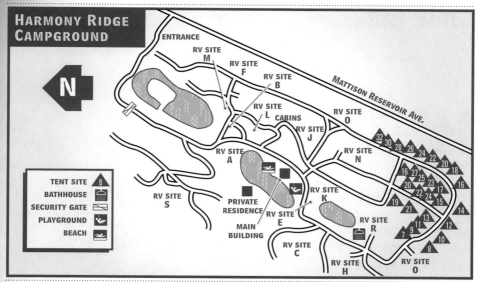

HARMONY RIDGE CAMPGROUND

N

ENTRANCE

RV SITE M
RV SITE F
RV SITE B
RV SITE L
CABINS
RV SITE O
RV SITE J
RV SITE A
RV SITE N
RV SITE S
RV SITE K
PRIVATE RESIDENCE
RV SITE E
RV SITE R
MAIN BUILDING
RV SITE C
RV SITE H
RV SITE O

MATTISON RESERVOIR AVE.

TENT SITE
BATHHOUSE
SECURITY GATE
PLAYGROUND
BEACH

GETTING THERE

From I-80, take Exit 34B (NJ 15 North). After 17.8 miles, NJ 15 becomes US 206. Continue north on US 206 to milepost 118. Turn right onto Ridge Road. At the end of Ridge Road, go left for 1 block to Mattison Reservoir Avenue. Go right on Mattison Reservoir Avenue for 1 mile. The campground entrance is on the left.

not enough. Only a few private campgrounds are able to satisfy both outdoorsy people and those looking for activities and structure. Harmony Ridge, with its idyllic setting on the Kittatinny Ridge, is the perfect home base for families who want to explore nearby Tillman Ravine, High Point State Park, or Stokes State Forest while still keeping Fido in tow and giving children some community recreation at the same time.

HIGH POINT STATE PARK

HIGH **POINT STATE PARK** sits at the top of New Jersey. Its 1,803-foot-tall mountain is the state's highest, and the park sits in the northernmost tip of the state, with the closest interstate in New York. The nearest large town is Port Jervis, a New York state town that sits 4 miles away at the junction of New York, New Jersey, and Pennsylvania. Port Jervis, long a transportation and rail center, has a commuter train that makes daily 90-minute trips to New York City. Campers wishing to tour Manhattan can use this train for day visits to New York City, while city dwellers can use this train in combination with taxi services to access the Appalachian Trail.

High Point's camping area is not near the contact station near Lake Marcia; that's the swimming and day-use area. The campground sits farther north up NJ 23, off Sawmill Road. Many sites are open, especially those right on Sawmill Lake, but there is plenty of space between these sections of prime real estate. You might see your neighbors at High Point State Park, but they won't be near enough to chat with.

Sites 46 through 50 are particularly appealing as they lie secluded at the end of the loop. They are set back in the woods, like the other sites on the outer loop. Some are not level, but large wooden tent platforms have been built. Some sites directly on the lake are walk-in, but the walks are too short to be of consequence to those carrying standard tent-camping gear. Remember, your cooler must always remain in your car in bear country, so consider the number of walks you'll make to the car when choosing a site. Only a few sites at Sawmill Lake are large enough for trailers, and there are no hookups or dump stations. Two rental cabins on the eastern shore of Steenykill Lake are available May through October.

Sawmill Lake is one of three public lakes at High

> *You might see your neighbors in this tent campground, but they won't be close enough to chat with.*

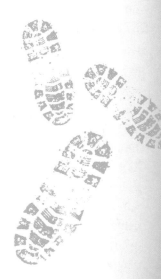

RATINGS

Beauty: ✿ ✿ ✿ ✿
Privacy: ✿ ✿ ✿
Spaciousness: ✿ ✿
Quiet: ✿ ✿
Security: ✿ ✿
Cleanliness: ✿ ✿ ✿

ADDRESS: High Point State
Park
1480 NJ 23
Sussex, NJ 07461

OPERATED BY: State Park Service

INFORMATION: (973) 875-4800

WEB SITE: www.njparksand
forests.org

OPEN: April–October

SITES: 50

EACH SITE HAS: Picnic table, fire ring

ASSIGNMENT: Choose from
available sites

REGISTRATION: On arrival or
reserve minimum 2
nights

FACILITIES: Water, flush toilets

PARKING: At site, maximum 2
vehicles

FEE: $15

ELEVATION: 1,300 feet

RESTRICTIONS: Pets: Prohibited
Fires: In fire rings
only
Alcohol: Prohibited
Vehicles: None; tents
only
Other: Quiet hours
10 p.m.–6 a.m.; 14-
night, 6-person, and
2-tent limit

Point. No swimming is allowed in Sawmill or Steenykill lakes, but you can launch boats from ramps at both. Only electric motors and nonmotorized boats are allowed. Fishing with a license is permitted in all three lakes, although boats are prohibited in Lake Marcia. Sawmill is stocked with trout, and all three lakes are home to perch, bass, catfish, and sunfish. Fishing licenses are available at some nearby businesses; check with the park office for details. There are no canoe concessions within High Point State Park, but three private firms rent canoes on the nearby Delaware River.

Spring-fed Lake Marcia offers the only swimming area at High Point. The sandy beach, along with its bathhouse and food concession, is open in summer when lifeguards are on duty. There are no trashcans at Lake Marcia. Visitors are given plastic bags at the contact station and are required to carry out all garbage. This not only contributes to a cleaner park but also reduces conflicts between wildlife and trash.

You'll have access to 11 official trails in 14,218-acre High Point State Park, in addition to an 18-mile stretch of the Appalachian Trail (A.T.). Campers can hike to the A.T. via the rugged 0.4-mile Blue Dot Trail.

Monument Trail is a popular 3.7-mile hiking loop that connects the day-use area to High Point Monument. The 220-foot-high granite obelisk, built in 1928, is a memorial to veterans and marks the highest point in New Jersey. The area around the monument offers sweeping vistas of the nearby mountains and can easily be reached by car from Monument Drive, but the hiking trail offers unique views of the three surrounding states of New York, New Jersey, and Pennsylvania. Most of the trail is uphill and was built in the 1930s by FDR's Civilian Conservation Corps. The Appalachian Trail does not go by High Point Monument, but A.T. hikers can detour to the monument via Scenic Drive and Monument Trail.

Part of Monument Trail crosses Cedar Swamp Natural Area, the highest elevated swamp of its kind in the world, within the 800-acre Dryden Kuser National Area. Pick up a booklet at park headquarters to take a self-guided nature walk along the bog trail.

Mountain biking and horseback riding are allowed

MAP

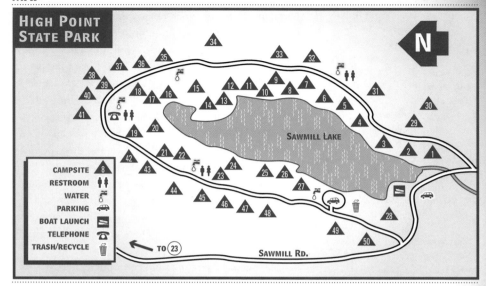

on eight of High Point's trails. Additionally, some trails allow cross-country skiing, dogsledding, and snowmobiling in winter. High Point Cross Country Ski Center opens during winter months and provides winter sports equipment rental as well as hot food. Artificial snow is manufactured for many of the trails.

High Point is not only the highest point in New Jersey, it is also one of the state's most rural and scenic spots. Don't miss the trip to the crest of the Kittatinny Ridge, even if you don't camp at placid Sawmill Lake.

GETTING THERE

From I-287, take Exit 52 and go north for 35 miles on NJ 23. From I-84, take Exit 1 and go south for 4 miles on NJ 23.

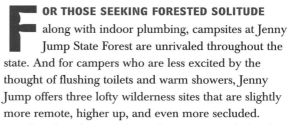

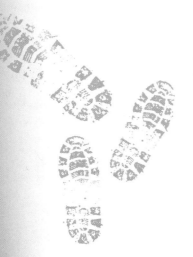

> *Private, wooded, lofty sites along with modern plumbing make Jenny Jump unrivaled throughout the state.*

FOR THOSE SEEKING FORESTED SOLITUDE along with indoor plumbing, campsites at Jenny Jump State Forest are unrivaled throughout the state. And for campers who are less excited by the thought of flushing toilets and warm showers, Jenny Jump offers three lofty wilderness sites that are slightly more remote, higher up, and even more secluded.

Developed sites at Jenny Jump are mostly level clearings, well spaced from each other, and encircled by trees and understory. Nine sites are designated walk-in, but six of these require only brief walks from parking areas. These six sites (22, 23, 26, 27, 34, 35) are located in the main camping area along East Road, close to restrooms and trails.

Campers will find the three wilderness sites in the woods above the eight rental cabins. You must carry your gear up a hill to the primitive sites, but the rustic perch is worth the effort. Sites offer no plumbing but do provide a gentle breeze on all but the warmest of days. Modern restrooms are located down the hill by the cabins, but hiking along the rocky path is not recommended after dark.

The terrain in Jenny Jump State Forest was gouged out 21,000 years ago at the end of the Wisconsin Ice Age. Advancing glaciers halted a few miles away, leaving debris and sediment, and carving out chunks of rock. The result was dramatic, leaving jagged boulders, rocky mountains, and valleys. Some of the man-made features can be attributed to the Civilian Conservation Corps (CCC), who built roads and the picnic area in the 1930s.

Other man-made features include a variety of legends and local folklore regarding the name of the road that goes to the Ghost Lake boat launch. The sinister tall tales that explain how Shades of Death Road and Ghost Lake were named run the gamut from the

RATINGS

Beauty: ✿ ✿ ✿ ✿ ✿
Privacy: ✿ ✿ ✿ ✿ ✿
Spaciousness: ✿ ✿ ✿
Quiet: ✿ ✿ ✿ ✿
Security: ✿ ✿ ✿
Cleanliness: ✿ ✿ ✿

believable (an 1850 malaria epidemic) to the absurd (a deerskin-bedecked Native American guards the road and will chase you). Jenny Jump itself has a disturbing legend behind its moniker; the myth claims that a girl named Jenny jumped off a cliff to avoid Native Americans in the 1700s. Park literature points out that it is just as likely that "Jenny Jump" is an anglicized version of a Lenape Native American name for the mountain. See the book *Weird N.J.* (Sceurman and Moran, 2004) for all the lurid legends surrounding the region.

Ghost Lake is famed more for its bass fishing opportunities than for its eeriness. Anglers can fish from small boats or canoes as well as from the shore. In addition to bass, crappie, sunfish, and catfish can also be caught in the shallow lake. Hunting is also permitted in some parts of Jenny Jump State Forest.

Faery Hole, a small cave, is accessible from the Ghost Lake dirt parking lot on Shades of Death Road. Look for a trail that goes up a rocky slope. The cave itself is simple and flat. All of its artifacts, including mammal bones and pottery, were excavated long ago.

Five short hiking trails, as well as the 3.7-mile Mount Lake multiuse trail, wind through the 4,200-acre forest. You can access Orchard, Swamp, Summit, and Spring trails from the camping area, while 1.3-mile Ghost Lake Trail meets East Road by the group camping area. The 1.5-mile Summit Trail climbs to 1,090 feet and offers panoramic vistas of the surrounding area. Hikers may encounter deer and turkey as well as a wide variety of birds. But keep your eyes on the ground as well. A number of snakes inhabit the forest.

On Saturday evenings between April and October, the United Astronomy Clubs of New Jersey offers public astronomy programs at their Jenny Jump observatory. The club's 16-inch Newtonian telescope is housed in leased state property that used to be a private home. The club chose Jenny Jump for its dark sky—one of the few dark spots left in the most densely populated state in the country.

For younger campers, commercial amusement park Land of Make Believe is nestled in the foothills of Jenny Jump State Forest. It offers a water park, carnival-style rides, and a small roller coaster. It's not

KEY INFORMATION

ADDRESS:	Jenny Jump State Forest P.O. Box 150 Hope, NJ 07844
OPERATED BY:	State Park Service
INFORMATION:	(908) 459-4366
WEB SITE:	www.njparksand forests.org
OPEN:	April–October
SITES:	22
EACH SITE HAS:	Picnic table, fire ring, lantern post (in developed sites)
ASSIGNMENT:	First come, first served
REGISTRATION:	On arrival or reserve minimum 2 nights
FACILITIES:	Water, flushing toilets, showers
PARKING:	Drive-in sites, 2-vehicle limit; walk-in sites, nearby lots
FEE:	$15
ELEVATION:	800 feet
RESTRICTIONS:	**Pets:** Prohibited **Fires:** In fire rings only **Alcohol:** Prohibited **Vehicles:** Up to 32 feet **Other:** Quiet hours 10 p.m.–6 a.m.; 14-night, 6-person, and 2-tent limit

MAP

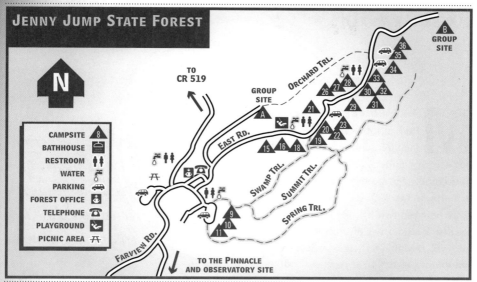

JENNY JUMP STATE FOREST

TO CR 519

GROUP SITE

GROUP SITE B

ORCHARD TRL.

N

CAMPSITE
BATHHOUSE
RESTROOM
WATER
PARKING
FOREST OFFICE
TELEPHONE
PLAYGROUND
PICNIC AREA

EAST RD.

SWAMP TRL.

SUMMIT TRL.

SPRING TRL.

FARVIEW RD.

TO THE PINNACLE
AND OBSERVATORY SITE

GETTING THERE

From I-80, take Exit 12. Take a slight left onto County Road 521 for 1.3 miles to the center of Hope. Turn left onto CR 519 at the blinking light. At the third right, turn onto Shiloh Road. After 1 mile, turn right onto State Park Road.

for those seeking adrenaline rides and is aimed at children ages 12 and younger. Rides include a turn-of-the-century carousel, a spinning tyrannosaurus rex, and waterslides. There's also a petting zoo and a participatory theater, where kids get to dress up and be part of a medieval show.

But the main attraction at Jenny Jump is the wilderness and the campground, not the local carnival. Reserve in advance in the summer—the cool, elevated sites under the trees go quickly.

MAHLON DICKERSON RESERVATION

MAHLON **D**ICKERSON **R**ESERVATION, best known for its multiuse trails, recreational facilities, and undeveloped wilderness areas, has the only public campground in Morris County. Surprisingly few people are aware of this rustic jewel of a campground, tucked away just north of Lake Hopatcong between two wildlife management areas in the northwestern corner of the county. Dogs on leashes are allowed at Mahlon Dickerson Reservation, a feature unique in a state where state parks do not allow pets in camping areas.

The eight tent sites are located on a dead-end single-track road—a spur that juts out from a loop dedicated to four shelters and a campfire ring. Two portable toilets and a dumpster are the only luxuries on offer, but a modern restroom with flushing toilets and hot showers is located a short drive away at the trailer area. (Restrooms are heated in the winter.) All sites offer 30- and 50-amp electrical hookups as well as water hookups in warmer months.

Tent sites are shaded and private, and most are mansions by camping standards. Not all sites are level, but each has a 12-by-12-foot flat wooden platform. Site 2 is wheelchair accessible.

For would-be campers who do not own tents, Mahlon Dickerson offers a limited number of rental tents as well as four shelters near the campfire ring. The shelters are popular in autumn and winter. Mahlon Dickerson's campsites are open year-round, but few people set up tents once ice-skating and cross-country skiing season begins.

Permits are required to camp at Mahlon Dickerson. Reserve ahead if possible, although sites are usually available on nonholiday weekdays and in off-season. Telephone reservations and credit cards are not accepted; to reserve ahead, send your payment

> *Mahlon Dickerson features plenty of accessible natural recreation close to an urban environment.*

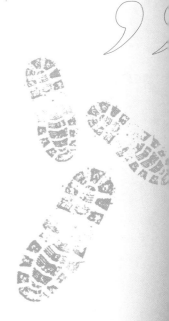

RATINGS

Beauty: ✩ ✩ ✩
Privacy: ✩ ✩ ✩ ✩
Spaciousness: ✩ ✩ ✩ ✩ ✩
Quiet: ✩ ✩ ✩ ✩
Security: ✩ ✩
Cleanliness: ✩ ✩

ADDRESS: Mahlon Dickerson
Reservation
P.O. Box 684
Lake Hopatcong, NJ
07849

OPERATED BY: Morris County Park
Commission

INFORMATION: (973) 663-0200

WEB SITE: www.morrisparks.net

OPEN: Year-round

SITES: 8

EACH SITE HAS: Picnic table, fire
ring, tent platform

ASSIGNMENT: Choose from
available sites

REGISTRATION: On arrival or by
reservation

FACILITIES: Vault and flush toilets, water, showers

PARKING: At sites or
designated lot

FEE: $10

ELEVATION: 1,100 feet

RESTRICTIONS: Pets: On leash
Fires: In fire rings by
permit only
Alcohol: Prohibited
Vehicles: Up to 35
feet
Other: Maximum
stay of 2 weeks in 30
days

and reservation by mail more than two weeks in advance. To register on arrival, go to the visitor center or campground office (May through October). After hours, register with the camp host at the trailer area or at the "quick registration" board at the entrance to the trailer area. If you have prepaid and reserved ahead, you may proceed straight to your campsite, which will be marked with your name and the date.

A multiuse trail starts from the cul-de-sac at the tent camping area, right beside site 8. Follow this path straight to the yellow trail (bike and foot traffic only), turning right to cut over to the teal-blazed Highlands Trail. To the left on the Highlands Trail are two view-points. Both offer panoramic views of the area, but the second one, Headley Overlook, is more popular as it is easier to access from Weldon Road.

The Highlands Trail, when completed, will tra-verse 150 miles between the Delaware River in Central New Jersey and the Hudson River in New York's Hud-son Valley. It is a cooperative conservation effort by state and local governments, local businesses, and the New York–New Jersey Trail Conference. The Mahlon Dickerson section enters the park in the south near NJ 15 and exits north of the trailer area.

Follow Highlands Trail north, crossing Weldon Road. From there, several trails branch off heading north or west. Find your way to the western section of Pine Swamp Trail to reach the highest point in Morris County at 1,395 feet.

The Morris County Park System prides itself on its dedication to multipurpose parks and spectacular set-tings. Nowhere is this more evident than at Mahlon Dickerson, where mountain bikers and equestrians are treated with the same consideration given to foot hik-ers. Mahlon Dickerson's 20 acres of multiuse trails include bike trails that are regarded as the best bike trails in Morris County, but they are not for beginners. Novices might consider practicing on the Morris County section of the Patriots Path, which is smoother. Mahlon Dickerson's mountain biking is technical with some steep climbs. The newest trail is a yellow-blazed 5.3-mile multiuse trail that begins at the Saffin Pond Area. Also popular is the 2.5-mile Edison Branch Rail

MAP

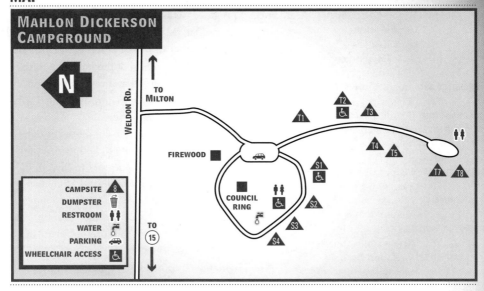

Trail, which follows an old rail trail. Trail maps are available at the Saffin Visitor Center and at information points around the park.

Saffin Pond features fishing and canoeing. For those who want to try more active watersports, Lake Hopatcong, with its waterskiing and swimming, is just a few miles away.

Only a small percentage of Mahlon Dickerson Reservation is developed. A hike or bike ride may take you past deer or beaver as well as many smaller mammals. With over 3,000 acres of near wilderness, Mahlon Dickerson features plenty of accessible natural recreation close to an urban environment.

GETTING THERE

From I-80, take NJ 15 north for 5 miles to Weldon Road. Go 4 miles on Weldon Road to the tent camping area on the right.

STEPHENS STATE PARK

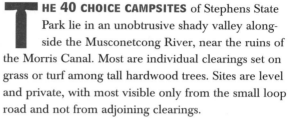

> *Visitors come to commune with nature, to fish, to boat, and to hike ruins of the Morris Canal.*

THE **40 CHOICE CAMPSITES** of Stephens State Park lie in an unobtrusive shady valley alongside the Musconetcong River, near the ruins of the Morris Canal. Most are individual clearings set on grass or turf among tall hardwood trees. Sites are level and private, with most visible only from the small loop road and not from adjoining clearings.

Eight of Stephens's campsites can accommodate small RVs, while three sites are large enough for 40-footers. As in most New Jersey state parks, no hookups are available. Only six sites are open; the remainder are forested. Many are small, but some can be combined with adjacent sites to form larger units. Use caution when camping on site 5, as it sometimes floods. Avoid sites 1, 2, 28, and 40 since they are next to the road. The campground at Stephens is wooded and feels rural, so avoid this reminder of civilization if at all possible.

There are no showers at this campground, but visitors do not come to Stephens for the bathhouses. They come to commune with nature, to hike the trails, to fish, and to boat. They come for the Morris Canal and Waterloo Village or to visit neighboring Alla-muchy Mountain State Park.

In the 1800s, the 102-mile-long Morris Canal was one of two major transportation arteries that brought anthracite coal east to New York City, returning goods west to Pennsylvania. The other canal, the Delaware and Raritan Canal, fared better than its sister—nearly the entire length of the D & R is now a New Jersey state park. By contrast, much of the Morris Canal was demolished. Parts of the former waterway form the bed of the Newark City Subway or the Hudson-Bergen Light Rail, and much of the right-of-way has been transformed into roads or utility lines. Some regional governments and citizens groups have recognized the

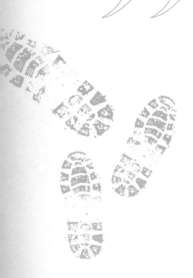

RATINGS

Beauty: ✰ ✰ ✰ ✰ ✰
Privacy: ✰ ✰ ✰ ✰
Spaciousness: ✰ ✰ ✰
Quiet: ✰ ✰ ✰ ✰ ✰
Security: ✰ ✰
Cleanliness: ✰ ✰ ✰

historic value of the "mountain-climbing canal," the route that overcame more elevation changes than any other similar canal in the world. Development has been halted in favor of preservation and greenways.

Lock 5 West sits at Saxton Falls, less than a mile upstream from Stephens State Park. The towpath alongside it is gradually being restored, and the publicly owned Allamuchy Mountain section of the towpath is the centerpiece for the canal trail, which hopefully will one day extend from Hackettstown to Ledgewood.

Other parts of the towpath have been preserved at Waterloo Village, a restored nineteenth-century Morris Canal town. Waterloo was an inland port that possessed one of the 23 inclined planes that made the Morris Canal a technological marvel. It is a National Historic Site and features a gristmill, sawmill, blacksmith shop, church, school, tavern, and inn. But the boom years of the Morris Canal are not the only ones featured. Revolutionary War–era buildings share space with Lenape Native American huts, in addition to structures from the Morris Canal heyday.

Saxton Falls is not just recommended for history buffs; it is also popular with anglers. On the first day of trout season, the scene has been described as "mayhem," but it's calm on other days. The Musconetcong (or "Musky") waters are stocked annually with brown, rainbow, and brook trout. Rock bass and sunfish are present in addition to trout, and the occasional eel is caught. In Allamuchy Mountain State Park, largemouth bass, sunfish, perch, and pickerel can be found in the lakes and ponds. Parts of Allamuchy Mountain State Park are open for hunting, subject to the rules and regulations of the New Jersey Division of Fish and Wildlife. Half of 805-acre Stephens is designated "no hunting."

Six miles of marked trails crisscross Stephens State Park, including a two-mile section of the Highlands Trail. When complete, the Highlands Trail will connect the Delaware River in New Jersey with the Hudson River in New York State. Allamuchy Mountain State Park features 15 miles of trails within the Allamuchy Natural Area, as well as an additional 25 miles of

KEY INFORMATION

ADDRESS: Stephens State Park 800 Willow Grove Street Hackettstown, NJ 07840

OPERATED BY: State Park Service

INFORMATION: (908) 852-3790

WEB SITE: www.njparksand forests.org

OPEN: April–October

SITES: 40

EACH SITE HAS: Picnic table, fire ring, lantern post

ASSIGNMENT: First come, first served

REGISTRATION: On arrival or reserve minimum 2 nights

FACILITIES: Water, flush toilets

PARKING: At site, 2-vehicle limit

FEE: $15

ELEVATION: 600 feet

RESTRICTIONS: Pets: Prohibited Fires: In fire rings only Alcohol: Prohibited Vehicles: Up to 40 feet Other: Quiet hours 10 p.m.–6 a.m.; 14-day, 6-person, and 2 tent limit

MAP

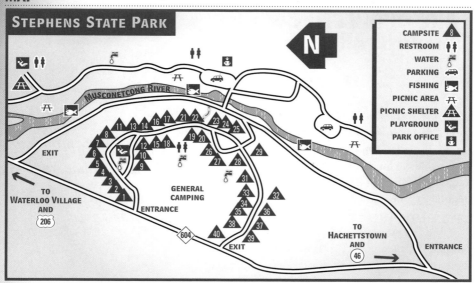

STEPHENS STATE PARK

N

CAMPSITE	8
RESTROOM	♗♗
WATER	
PARKING	
FISHING	
PICNIC AREA	🛇
PICNIC SHELTER	🛆
PLAYGROUND	
PARK OFFICE	

MUSCONETCONG RIVER

EXIT

TO
WATERLOO VILLAGE
AND
206

GENERAL
CAMPING

ENTRANCE

604

EXIT

TO
HACHETTSTOWN
AND
46

ENTRANCE

GETTING THERE

From I-80, travel north on US 206 for 1.3 miles. Turn left onto Willow Grove Street (County Road 604). Drive 7.5 miles to the campground entrance, on the left.

unmarked trails in the park's northern section. Trails within both parks are designated multiuse and can be used by hikers, equestrians, and cyclists, although some trails are rocky. One 3-mile trail is designated a water trail and follows the Musconetcong River from Waterloo Road to the Saxton Falls Dam.

Stephens is well known for its interpretive nature programs. On weekends and holidays, rangers and naturalists present educational workshops on many topics including ecology, trees, insects, owls, orienteering, bears, camping safety, and the culture of the Lenape Native Americans. Programs are popular with older children as well as with adults.

STOKES STATE FOREST LAKE OCQUITTUNK CAMPING AREA

MORE SCENIC THAN Shotwell Camping Area but less rustic than Steam Mill, Lake Ocquittunk Camping Area provides the best of both worlds in Stokes State Forest, combining a remote natural lifestyle with top-notch modern plumbing facilities. Sites are spread throughout three areas, with a separate section dedicated to cabin camping.

Most picturesque is Big Flatbrook Loop. Sites 15 through 19 sit along the pleasantly bubbling creek. Sites are private, near restrooms, and sit under tall hardwoods. Sites 13 and 14 are isolated at the other end of the brook. Both have tent platforms, and while they lack restrooms, they offer total seclusion. Sites 1 through 12 are on the entry road and closest to the showers. Cabins are on a separate loop; linens and cooking utensils are not provided. Prices for cabins range from $28 to $70 per night.

Some anglers have called Big Flatbrook one of New Jersey's finest rivers. It's really more a creek than a river, and the tumbling of water over rocks fills the river with oxygen. The river and lake are both stocked with trout, but other fish call them home too. Only fish are allowed to swim in Big Flatbrook and eight-acre Lake Ocquittunk, although boating is allowed. People must drive or hike to the day-use area at Stony Lake to swim. Swimming is permitted there in summer when a lifeguard is on duty.

Two dozen trails crisscross Stokes State Forest. Blue Mountain Trail, an easy 1.4-mile route, is the closest trail to the campground. It links up with Kittle Road to provide you with a hiking or bicycle route to the swimming area at Stony Lake. Tinsley Trail heads southeast from the campground for 2.8 miles and offers a challenging hike up to the Appalachian Trail.

For some scenic walks that are not on the trail map, take a ride over to Tillman Ravine, at the most

> *Set up camp alongside what some anglers call one of New Jersey's finest rivers.*

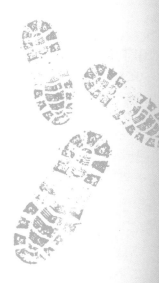

RATINGS

Beauty: ✪ ✪ ✪ ✪
Privacy: ✪ ✪ ✪
Spaciousness: ✪ ✪ ✪
Quiet: ✪ ✪ ✪ ✪
Security: ✪ ✪
Cleanliness: ✪ ✪ ✪

ADDRESS:	Stokes State Forest 1 Coursen Road Branchville, NJ 07826
OPERATED BY:	State Park Service
INFORMATION:	(973) 948-3820
WEB SITE:	www.njparksand forests.org
OPEN:	April–October
SITES:	24
EACH SITE HAS:	Picnic table, fire ring
ASSIGNMENT:	First come, first served
REGISTRATION:	On arrival or reserve minimum 2 nights
FACILITIES:	Water, flush toilets, showers
PARKING:	At site, maximum 2 vehicles
FEE:	$15
ELEVATION:	700 feet
RESTRICTIONS:	**Pets:** Prohibited **Fires:** In fire rings only **Alcohol:** Prohibited **Vehicles:** Up to 24 feet **Other:** Quiet hours 10 p.m.–6 a.m.; 14-night, 6-person, and 2-tent limit; no gas motors or swimming in Lake Ocquittunk

southwestern point of Stokes State Forest. Follow the park map to get there or just head west on Strubble Road off US 206. Leave your car in the parking lot and follow the trail into the evergreens. Tillman Brook carves the ravine out of sandstone and shale as it descends from the Kittatinny Ridge. When it hits the bottom of the ravine, the water creates a bowl-like area, nicknamed the "Teacup." Hikers like to relax under the forest canopy, put their feet into the cold waters of the pothole, and watch the brook cascade down the hill. Note that there are no facilities at Tillman Ravine.

A pleasant waterfall, Buttermilk Falls, is near Tillman Ravine. Exit the parking lot to the left on Brink Road and continue to dirt Mountain Road. Go left for 2 miles to Buttermilk Falls. If you stay on Brink Road just a little longer, you will enter Walpack Center. Almost a ghost town now, Walpack Center was a thriving farming community over a hundred years ago. Today it is a designated historic district that is slowly being restored by volunteers from the Walpack Historical Society and the National Park Service. Many old buildings in the region were destroyed during the planning stages for a massive dam that was to be built on the Delaware River. Local residents fought the dam in the 1970s, but many buildings had already been destroyed by the time the project was abandoned. Eleven buildings in the village center survived.

Just north of Walpack Center is the Walpack Inn, an acclaimed restaurant. The sign out front declares that they feed deer as well as people, and the dining room looks out over lush green fields where deer often snack.

Continue northeast on County Road 615 for 3.2 miles and you will reach the Kuhn Road turnoff for Peters Valley Craft Education Center. The center is dedicated to craft education in several disciplines: blacksmithing, ceramics, fine metals, photography, surface design, weaving, and woodworking. Additional special topics such as wearable art, mosaic design, and culinary sculpture are sometimes added. The on-site store and gallery is open Friday through Wednesday, 11 a.m. to 5 p.m. and features work by local and national artists. Additionally, the center has a craft fair

MAP

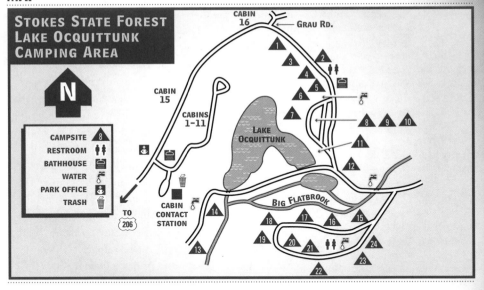

STOKES STATE FOREST LAKE OCQUITTUNK CAMPING AREA

N

CAMPSITE	8
RESTROOM	♀♂
BATHHOUSE	🚿
WATER	🚰
PARK OFFICE	🏢
TRASH	🗑

CABIN 16

GRAU RD.

CABIN 15

CABINS 1–11

LAKE OCQUITTUNK

BIG FLATBROOK

TO 206

CABIN CONTACT STATION

once a year and hosts occasional open houses, lectures, and presentations.

Creekside spots at Lake Ocquittunk Camping Area are some of the nicest sites in the region, so call ahead for summer weekends. Remember to bring your fishing pole, hiking boots, and a map of regional attractions.

GETTING THERE

From I-80, take Exit 34B to NJ 15 North. After 18 miles, NJ 15 becomes US 206 North. After 6.7 miles, turn right onto Coursen Road at the top of the mountain to pay for camping at the visitor center. Exit back onto US 206, going right for 2 miles to Flatbrook Road. Turn right and drive 3 miles to the campground entrance on the right.

STOKES STATE FOREST SHOTWELL CAMPING AREA

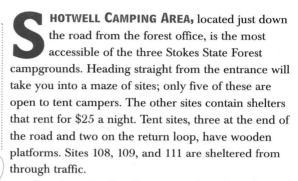

> *Stokes's inaccessibility prior to the completion of I-80 preserved it from development for hundreds of years.*

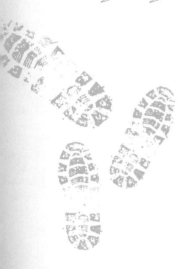

SHOTWELL **CAMPING AREA,** located just down the road from the forest office, is the most accessible of the three Stokes State Forest campgrounds. Heading straight from the entrance will take you into a maze of sites; only five of these are open to tent campers. The other sites contain shelters that rent for $25 a night. Tent sites, three at the end of the road and two on the return loop, have wooden platforms. Sites 108, 109, and 111 are sheltered from through traffic.

Four tent sites line the one-way loop in and out of the campground, but the best tent sites are on the spur road that veers left off the main thoroughfare. These spacious sites are more secluded, rustic, and offer a semblance of privacy. Sites 131 through 135 sit on a grassy field and require a brief walk from a central parking area. All sites have lantern posts in addition to picnic tables and fire rings, and some are situated on pleasant Shotwell Pond (no swimming allowed). Campers at the end of the spur will have to take hearty walks to reach the flush toilets.

Stokes State Forest and the surrounding area were considered remote prior to the completion of I-80 in the 1970s. Its inaccessibility preserved it from development back in 1907, when the first 5,000 acres were purchased by the state of New Jersey and added to 500 acres bequeathed by Edward C. Stokes, then governor of New Jersey. The governor's greatest legacy was not in providing stiffer penalties for Sunday liquor sales but in creating water and forest commissions. Today, Stokes State Forest covers 15,947 acres, including 2,900 acres recently added through New Jersey's public Green Acres Program.

Nine of the Appalachian Trail's 2,000 miles cut through Stokes State Forest. Those who dream of being thru-hikers can test their mettle on the 5-mile

RATINGS

Beauty: ✿ ✿ ✿ ✿
Privacy: ✿ ✿ ✿
Spaciousness: ✿ ✿ ✿
Quiet: ✿ ✿ ✿ ✿
Security: ✿ ✿ ✿
Cleanliness: ✿ ✿ ✿

walk from US 206 to Sunrise Mountain. Follow the white blazes and pretend you've been walking for months.

Three shelters provide camping for hikers on A.T. trips that require overnight stops, but day hikers must use one of the three developed campgrounds within Stokes. The Ladder, Acropolis, Tower, Stony Brook, Tinsley, Cartwright, and Howell trails, as well as Sunrise Mountain Road, provide access to the Appalachian Trail from Stokes. A parking lot at Sunrise Mountain offers vehicle access to this 1,653-foot perch. To the east are the Jersey Highlands, and to the west are the Poconos. The rolling hills of Sussex County lie all around. The pavilion at the summit is a remnant of the Civilian Conservation Corps work from the 1930s. The area is popular with birders, particularly in late August and September.

For a short geology lesson, follow Tinsley Trail from Sunrise Mountain Road to the Kittatinny Glacial Geology Trail. This self-guided trail is short and easy, although a little rocky in places. Fifteen numbered posts along the way correspond to numbered paragraphs in the trail brochure, which explains how the region transformed into the Kittatinny Ridge over the years after being a vast inland seacoast.

A colorful exhibit at the forest office reminds campers that lantern posts are for lanterns, not for food. Some campers have hung food from posts instead of storing it in their cars with the windows rolled up or in bear-proof containers. Bears smell the food and linger at campsites, trying to reach it. Often they do reach it, as the lantern posts are not the recommended 12 feet from the ground. Remember, bears live in the area, so always use bear-proof containers and never take food into or near your tent. See the Introduction for more information on how to camp safely in bear country.

Both a 4-H camp and a Boy Scout camp are located due west of Shotwell Camping Area; neither is open to the public. Stony Lake in the day-use area is, however, open to campers. Swimming is allowed in Stony Lake during summer, provided lifeguards are on

KEY INFORMATION

ADDRESS:	Stokes State Forest 1 Coursen Road Branchville, NJ 07826
OPERATED BY:	State Park Service
INFORMATION:	(973) 948-3820
WEB SITE:	www.njparksand forests.org
OPEN:	Year-round
SITES:	27
EACH SITE HAS:	Picnic table, fire ring
ASSIGNMENT:	First come, first served
REGISTRATION:	On arrival or reserve minimum 2 nights
FACILITIES:	Water, flush toilets
PARKING:	At site, 2-vehicle limit
FEE:	$15
ELEVATION:	800 feet
RESTRICTIONS:	Pets: Prohibited Fires: In fire rings only Alcohol: Prohibited Vehicles: Up to 24 feet; no hookups Other: Quiet hours 10 p.m.–6 a.m.; 14-night, 6-person, 2-tent limit; no tents allowed on lean-to sites; no swimming in Shotwell Pond

MAP

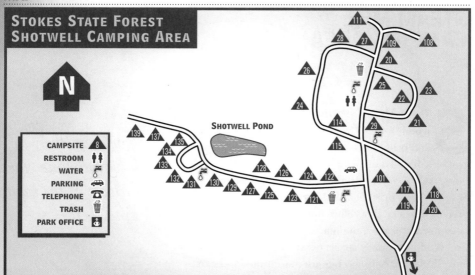

STOKES STATE FOREST SHOTWELL CAMPING AREA

N

SHOTWELL POND

CAMPSITE	8
RESTROOM	♀♂
WATER	🚰
PARKING	🚗
TELEPHONE	☎
TRASH	🗑
PARK OFFICE	👤

GETTING THERE

From I-80, take Exit 34B to NJ 15 North. After 18 miles, NJ 15 becomes US 206 North. After 6.7 miles, turn right onto Coursen Road at the top of the mountain. Follow the signs from the visitor center to Shotwell Campground.

duty. A food concession operates when the swimming beach is open. The bathhouse and CCC-constructed picnic area with grills and a pavilion are always open. Fishing is allowed in Stony Lake, and there is a playground nearby. For people who enjoy the outdoors, there's something for everyone at Stokes State Forest.

STOKES STATE FOREST STEAM MILL CAMPING AREA

STEAM MILL CAMPING AREA, set back in the woods 5 miles from US 206, is the most remote and primitive of the Stokes State Forest campgrounds. It's also the least patronized one, and the most likely to have a site even during high season. Sites are wide-open with little or no foliage to act as privacy barriers. But you're unlikely to have many neighbors, at least of the human kind.

Wildlife casually strolls nearby as you set up your tent. Trailers fit here too but are more suited to Lake Ocquittunk. Remember, bears live in the area, so use bear-proof containers and never take food into or near your tent. See the Introduction for more information on how to camp safely in bear country.

The nearest neighbor to Steam Mill is a former Civilian Conservation Camp built in the 1930s by FDR's "army with shovels." One of FDR's first acts as president was to create a system of camps that employed young men in rural conservation projects. Today the camp's residents have similar goals, as the New Jersey School of Conservation has taken up residency on the 240-acre property.

The New Jersey School of Conservation, run by Montclair State University, is the oldest university-operated environmental education center in the nation. It became an environmental education center in 1949 but did not become state-operated until 1972. In addition to offering programs in environmental science and ecology, it offers astronomical research at its observatory and short environmental workshops for elementary and secondary school students. Gifted young musicians attend a two-week workshop in music ecology in the summer, and young adults attend fly-fishing classes on the 12-acre lake.

Stokes State Forest is a hiker's dream destination, with more than 40 miles of trails. Fall is a great time to

> *You're unlikely to have many neighbors, at least of the human kind, here.*

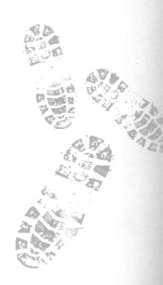

RATINGS

Beauty: ✿ ✿ ✿ ✿
Privacy: ✿ ✿
Spaciousness: ✿ ✿ ✿
Quiet: ✿ ✿ ✿
Security: ✿ ✿
Cleanliness: ✿ ✿

ADDRESS:	Stokes State Forest 1 Coursen Road Branchville, NJ 07826
OPERATED BY:	State Park Service
INFORMATION:	(973) 948-3820
WEB SITE:	www.njparksand forests.org
OPEN:	April–October
SITES:	26
EACH SITE HAS:	Picnic table, fire ring
ASSIGNMENT:	First come, first served
REGISTRATION:	On arrival or reserve minimum 2 nights
FACILITIES:	Water, vault toilets
PARKING:	At site, 2-vehicle limit
FEE:	$15
ELEVATION:	800 feet
RESTRICTIONS:	Pets: Prohibited Fires: In fire rings only Alcohol: Prohibited Vehicles: Up to 24 feet Other: Quiet hours 10 p.m.–6 a.m.; 14-night, 6-person, and 2-tent limit

visit—the foliage is turning color, and bears are wandering around hunting food as they fatten up for their winter hibernation.

Parker Trail begins right across from Steam Mill Camping Area and follows Parker Brook for 2.3 miles through neighboring High Point State Park. Its winding hills are classified as moderately difficult. Parker Brook is a wild trout stream. Anglers planning on fishing in Parker Brook should familiarize themselves with New Jersey fishing regulations, as certain wild trout restrictions are in effect year-round.

The Appalachian Trail and the dramatic panorama from 1,600-foot Sunrise Mountain are less than 2 miles from the campground. The most direct route, the Cartwright Trail, is classified as difficult. It rises dramatically over 0.9 miles, but seasoned hikers will make relatively short work of its winding slopes. Be aware that the streambed running along the path is not the trail. Cartwright Trail can be accessed from Swenson Trail off Sunrise Mountain Road. Turn right from the campground, or you could walk along the road for the entire distance. Driving to Sunrise Mountain is tempting, but Sunrise Mountain Road is one-way from US 206 to the campground—in the wrong direction.

Swenson Trail offers a moderate 3.8-mile hike at an elevation of 1,000 feet through a rocky ravine and several streams. The reward is the swimming and day-use area at Stony Lake, which lies at the end of the trail. From Sunrise Mountain, it is also possible to follow the A.T. to the Tower Trail, where you can get a view of the surrounding area if the fire tower is unmanned, before descending to Stony Lake.

The less ambitious can take an easy walk along 0.8-mile Steam Mill Trail. This route ends at the conservation school, where a road continues to Lake Ocquittunk. From there, it is possible to circle back around to Steam Mill Camping Area by following the mostly level road.

Steam Mill is designated a carry in/carry out area. Remove your trash, leaving it in bear-proof dumpsters at the cabin contact station by Lake Ocquittunk. Drive carefully as you leave—bears, chipmunks, turkeys, and deer are used to having the right-of-way.

MAP

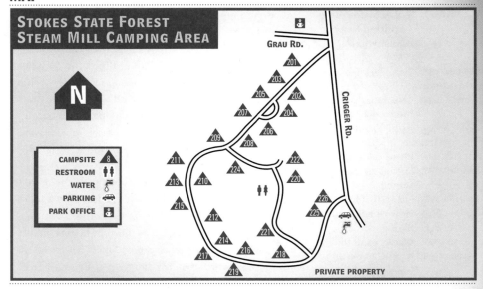

STOKES STATE FOREST
STEAM MILL CAMPING AREA

GRAU RD.

CRIGGER RD.

N

CAMPSITE	8
RESTROOM	👫
WATER	🚰
PARKING	🚗
PARK OFFICE	🏢

201
203
205 202
207 204
209 206
208

211 222
224 220
213 210

215 226
212 225

214 221
217 216 218
219

PRIVATE PROPERTY

GETTING THERE

From I-80, take Exit 34B to NJ 15 North. After 18 miles, NJ 15 becomes US 206 North. After 6.7 miles, turn right onto Coursen Road at the top of the mountain to pay for camping at the visitor center. Exit and turn right back onto US 206 North for 2 miles to Flatbrook Road. Turn right and drive 5 miles to the end of the road. Turn right to the campground entrance.

SWARTSWOOD STATE PARK

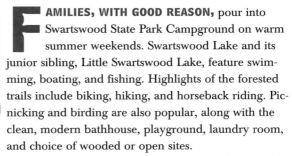

> *Freshwater Swartswood Lake has been a resort area since the 1900s.*

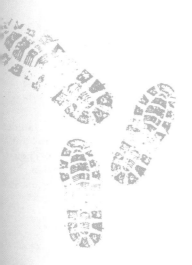

FAMILIES, WITH GOOD REASON, pour into Swartswood State Park Campground on warm summer weekends. Swartswood Lake and its junior sibling, Little Swartswood Lake, feature swimming, boating, and fishing. Highlights of the forested trails include biking, hiking, and horseback riding. Picnicking and birding are also popular, along with the clean, modern bathhouse, playground, laundry room, and choice of wooded or open sites.

The grassy open sites are larger and closer to the bathhouse. Choose them if you want to sacrifice privacy for space and community. They're popular with families and groups who want to stay in adjacent areas. The sites closest to the campground entrance will have constant traffic rolling by, so use caution when setting up camp near the entrance.

Two wooded loops are set against forested areas, where the tangled understory gives an illusion of privacy. Sites are spacious for one large tent, but some can become cramped if two tents are set up. The small one-way roads can be filled with children on bicycles. Children should wear helmets as required by New Jersey state law. A boat launch for campers only is directly across from site 37.

Six yurts are set off on a loop by themselves. They have their own bathhouse, which might be worth the walk if you get tired of waiting for the shower on the main loop.

The two glacial lakes have had problems with silt and plant growth. A watershed management program involving hungry weevils was put into place, with the end result being a safe and clean lake that appeals to both swimmers and fish. The protected swimming beach is across the park entrance road from the campground, but campers can also reach it via a lakeside multiuse trail. Lifeguards staff the beach from Memorial

RATINGS

Beauty: ✿ ✿ ✿
Privacy: ✿ ✿
Spaciousness: ✿ ✿ ✿
Quiet: ✿ ✿
Security: ✿ ✿
Cleanliness: ✿ ✿ ✿

Day weekend to Labor Day. It is closed when no life-guards are on duty. Facilities include a refreshment stand, first-aid room, and a bathhouse.

Swartswood is famed for its fishing opportunities. Both freshwater lakes are stocked with trout in the spring, and other fish are present throughout the year. Swartswood has been called one of the best walleye spots in New Jersey and is sometimes known as a great largemouth bass spot, but anglers have occasionally complained about the size of the lake, the wind, and the rule that powerboats are limited to electric motors. At around 500 acres of surface water, Swartswood Lake is one of the largest natural lakes in the state. Most of it is over 10 feet deep (over 50 feet deep near Pike Rock).

In addition to electric powerboats, small privately owned watercraft may be launched from three free public ramps. Rowboats, canoes, paddleboats, kayaks, and small sailboats can be rented at the park from a concessionaire near the swimming area. Parking is limited by the boat launch areas, but there is plenty of parking by the swimming beach. You must wear a life jacket when boating or sailing.

Four miles of multiuse trails begin across East Shore Drive from the entrance. First is the 0.6-mile-long Duck Pond Trail, a paved path accessible to wheelchairs, strollers, skateboards, cyclists, and skaters. The path features a bird blind as well as exhibits that explain natural features along the route. Branching off at the southern end of the Duck Pond is the 2.8-mile moderately difficult Spring Lake Trail. Follow it through varied forest habitats before passing both Spring Lake and Frog Pond and then looping back to Duck Pond. Follow 0.8-mile Bear Claw Trail for an easier option. Because hunting is allowed, be cautious and wear bright clothes in this section during hunting season.

Hikers can reach 1.5-mile Grist Mill Trail from the southwestern end of the lake, near the dam area off West Shore Drive (Route 521). It is not accessible from the campground without transportation. Grist Mill Trail is difficult but rewards hikers with views of the lake. Keen's Grist Mill, at the tip of the lake, was built in 1838 on the site of earlier mills.

KEY INFORMATION

ADDRESS:	Swartswood State Park P.O. Box 123 Swartswood, NJ 07877
OPERATED BY:	State Park Service
INFORMATION:	(973) 383-5230
WEB SITE:	www.njparksandforests.org
OPEN:	April–October
SITES:	65
EACH SITE HAS:	Picnic table, fire ring, lantern post
ASSIGNMENT:	First come, first served
REGISTRATION:	On arrival or reserve minimum 2 nights
FACILITIES:	Water, flush toilets, showers
PARKING:	At site, 2-vehicle limit
FEE:	$15
ELEVATION:	500 feet
RESTRICTIONS:	Pets: Prohibited Fires: In fire rings only Alcohol: Prohibited Vehicles: No limit Other: Quiet hours 10 p.m.–6 a.m.; 14-night, 6 person, and 2-tent limit

MAP

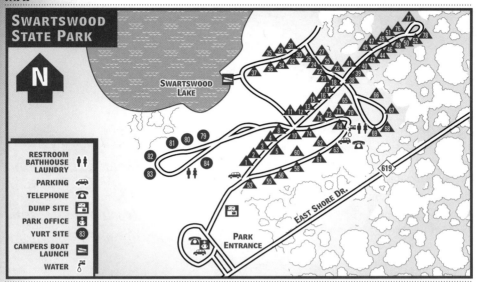

SWARTSWOOD STATE PARK

N

SWARTSWOOD LAKE

RESTROOM BATHHOUSE LAUNDRY	👫
PARKING	🚗
TELEPHONE	☎
DUMP SITE	🗑
PARK OFFICE	🛈
YURT SITE	83
CAMPERS BOAT LAUNCH	⛵
WATER	🚰

EAST SHORE DR.

619

PARK ENTRANCE

GETTING THERE

From I-80, take US 206 north to Newton. In Newton, turn left onto County Road 519 for half a mile. Turn left onto CR 622 for 5.3 miles. Go left onto CR 619 for half a mile to the park entrance.

Swartswood Lake got its name from British Captain Anthony Swartout, who lived on the lake with his family in the 1700s. He incurred the wrath of Native Americans through his service during the French and Indian Wars. In 1756, Swartout was killed by some of his enemies. The lake became a weekend resort in the early 1900s, with the advent of the railroad through Blairstown. It is still a weekend retreat today, although visitors are more likely to stay in tents than in inns or boarding houses.

WORTHINGTON STATE FOREST

FOUR-AND-ONE-HALF MILLION people visit the Delaware Water Gap Recreation Area every year. Fortunately, these visitors spread out over 40 miles of river and 70,000 acres of land across two states. Still, reserve your campsite ahead of time on summer weekends because Worthington State Forest Campground offers the only public developed sites within the park's boundaries.

The campground stretches along the Delaware River for 2 miles and is situated just north of the Delaware Water Gap itself. Kittatinny Mountain, part of the Appalachian Range, rises above the camping area. Sites to the right of the central forest office are sunnier; most surround a treeless field. The 23 sites to the left of the office are prized by those who prefer shade to sun; they are situated under a tall forest. These sites offer understory between sites as well as spacious, level tent areas. Throughout the campground, sites close to the river are level. Sites on the grassy field are more suitable for trailers, but there are no hookups anywhere in the campground.

Worthington State Forest Campground offers some of the newest bathhouses in New Jersey, as well as plenty of fresh water and well-situated toilets. Three bathhouses include multiple shower facilities as well as bicycle racks and pay phones. Two playgrounds and a basketball court are nearby. All toilets near sites 29 through 77 are modern and flushable. Some toilets near sites 1 through 23 are primitive, although the main bathhouse is modern. There are vending machines next to the bathhouse by the entrance road; one contains drinks while the other serves up live fishing bait.

Seventy-two miles of the famed Appalachian Trail traverse New Jersey with 7.8 of those miles in Worthington State Forest. The scenic walk from the Delaware Water Gap to Worthington's Sunfish Pond

> *Worthington State Forest Campground offers the only public developed sites within the park's boundaries*

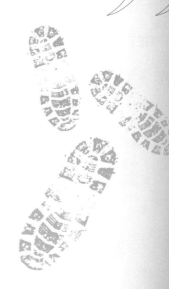

RATINGS

Beauty: ☆ ☆ ☆
Privacy: ☆ ☆ ☆
Spaciousness: ☆ ☆ ☆ ☆
Quiet: ☆ ☆ ☆
Security: ☆ ☆ ☆
Cleanliness: ☆ ☆ ☆ ☆

is the most popular section in the state and gets crowded on summer weekends. Ambitious campers can avoid the A.T. day-hiker crowds and hike up the 1.1-mile Turquoise Trail to Sunfish Pond. Unfortunately, while the most direct route provides pleasant views as it passes waterfalls and follows a bubbling creek, the Turquoise Trail rises 900 feet within a mile. Douglas Trail provides a 2.5-mile moderate alternative. It leaves from the campground and rises 900 feet over 2 miles before intersecting with the A.T. Follow the white blazes of the A.T. left to Sunfish Pond, passing the backpacker's campsite en route.

Sunfish Pond is a clear glacial lake formed during the last Ice Age. Hikers like to sit on its rocky shore for a rest or picnic lunch. Swimming in the lake is illegal, although the beavers don't seem to be aware of this restriction. Few fish live in the 41-acre lake; its acidic waters only support a few sturdy species.

You should remove all trash from Sunfish Pond and take it back to camp with you. All of Worthington State Forest is designated carry in/carry out. Bags are provided throughout the forest, and a dumpster is situated by the forest office at the entrance to the campground. This policy is not just about environmental responsibility; a large population of black bears live in the area. See the Introduction for more information on how to camp safely in bear country. Rattlesnakes and ticks also call the area home. Be prepared.

Other popular hikes go to Mohican Point at the northern end of the forest and Mount Tammany at the southern end. Both are renowned for their scenic vistas, outlooks that feature panoramic views of the surrounding region.

Fishing, hunting, and boating are also popular in Worthington. Some anglers have reported that the fishing off of Worthington is the best on the Delaware River. It is known for its spring shad run as well as its summer bass population. A small boat launch ramp is near the forest office, or campers can fish in waders or from the river's edge. Up on the Kittatinny Ridge, Dunnfield Creek is famed for its natural brook trout fishery. Special wild trout stream regulations apply.

MAP

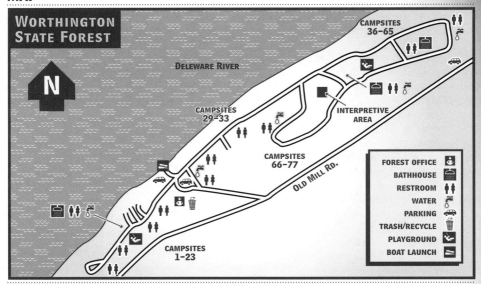

In the 1890s, millionaire Charles Worthington began purchasing land in the area. He bought 8,000 acres, including the village of Brotzmanville, where the campground sits today. He made much of it into a private preserve and reintroduced deer and pheasant, but he did not destroy the village. That happened later, during a 1955 flood. New Jersey began purchasing the land from Worthington's heirs in 1954. Today, Worthington's former home covers 6,200 wooded acres of land and features one of the most popular campgrounds on the Delaware River.

GETTING THERE

From I-80 at the NJ–PA border, take Exit 1 (Millbrook/Flatbrookville). Turn right at the bottom of the ramp onto Old Mill Road. Go north 3 miles to the office and campground on the left.

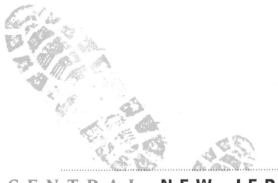

CENTRAL NEW JERSEY

IN 1822, businessman James P. Allaire headed south from Manhattan. He founded Howell Iron Works Company on an industrial bog iron processing area active since 1793. His integrated mining, smelting, and forging business thrived for a few decades, with more than 400 people living on company land during the 1830s. Howell Works' self-contained private community included homes, a church, a school, and service businesses such as a general store, blacksmith shop, carpenter's shop, and a bakery.

By the 1850s, bog furnaces were well on their way to extinction. Howell Works became a ghost town and was used as a movie studio, a French restaurant, and a Boy Scout camp before volunteers began restoration in the 1950s. Today Howell Works is called Allaire Village and is an outdoor living-history museum located within the confines of Allaire State Park.

Today's only residents of Allaire live in the campground for a maximum of two consecutive weeks. The tranquil campground is more than a mile away from the village and central activity area and consists of four small loops around a central bathhouse and playground.

The 45 sites can be used for tents or RVs, but the only concession to motorized camping is the dump station located near the entrance. There are no electrical or water hookups. There are, however, four yurts and six cabin-like shelters. These contain bunks and locking doors but no running water or electricity. Shelters feature woodstoves for those months when sleeping in a tent in the northeastern winter is unadvisable.

Tent sites are spacious, with varying degrees of privacy. Most are shaded, but there is little undergrowth or shrubbery between sites inside the loops. Try to get a site along the outer loop edges. All are within comfortable walking distance of the bathhouse and pay phone.

> *The roar of civilization seems far from the campground, although historic Allaire Village is only a mile away.*

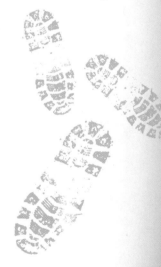

RATINGS

Beauty: ✿ ✿ ✿
Privacy: ✿ ✿
Spaciousness: ✿ ✿ ✿
Quiet: ✿ ✿ ✿
Security: ✿ ✿ ✿
Cleanliness: ✿ ✿ ✿

KEY INFORMATION

ADDRESS:	Allaire State Park P.O. Box 220 Farmingdale, NJ 07727
OPERATED BY:	New Jersey State Park Service
INFORMATION:	(732) 938-2371
WEB SITE:	www.njparksand forests.org
OPEN:	Year-round
SITES:	45; 10 yurt and shelter sites
EACH SITE HAS:	Picnic table, fire ring
ASSIGNMENT:	First come, first served
REGISTRATION:	On arrival or reserve minimum 2 nights
FACILITIES:	Water, flush toilets, showers
PARKING:	At site, 2-vehicle limit
FEE:	$15
ELEVATION:	50 feet
RESTRICTIONS:	Pets: Prohibited Fires: In fire rings only Alcohol: Prohibited Vehicles: No limit; no hookups Other: Quiet hours 10 p.m.–6 a.m.; 14-night, 6-person, and 2-tent limit

Allaire's campground is open year-round, but Allaire Village keeps seasonal hours. Most of the historic buildings are open Wednesday through Sunday during summer but only on weekends in fall. The General Store and Bakery open earlier in the season and stay open until December. Some holidays and weekends feature special events, such as hayrides, antique shows, or period-dress récreations. Call (732) 919-3500 to confirm opening hours.

The other man-made attraction within Allaire is the Pine Creek Railroad, New Jersey's only narrow-gauge preservation train. Pine Creek Railroad runs under its own steam on summer weekends and during the December holiday season but is diesel-powered in spring, fall, and on summer weekdays. Celebrities such as Santa Claus and the Easter Bunny have been known to join the crowds for the 10-minute 1.5-mile whirl around the park during holiday seasons.

The park also features more traditional offerings. Allaire's 3,086 acres include hiking, bridle, and biking trails along with opportunities for boating, fishing, and birding. The state-run Spring Meadow Golf Course is adjacent to the park. Cross-country skiing is allowed in winter, and limited deer hunting is allowed seasonally.

Much of the park has been left in its natural state as a habitat for wildlife and plants. Several trails wind through the forest, but when visiting, you are encouraged to stick to official blazed trails to avoid damaging both the environment and yourself (say, if you get bitten by a tick carrying Lyme Disease). So always stay on the trail and, in summer, do a full-body tick check after each foray into the woods.

Yellow, red, and green trails are easy trails designated for pedestrians only. The 16.5-mile-long orange-blazed trail is the official multiuse track, although some cyclists have complained that sand on the trail makes it less than appealing.

An easy ride begins just outside the park, where Hospital Road meets the abandoned Freehold-Jamesburg railroad right-of-way. Edgar Felix Bicycle Path is 5 miles long and goes to the center of the seaside town of Manasquan. It will eventually be part of New Jersey's "Capitol to the Coast" project that

MAP

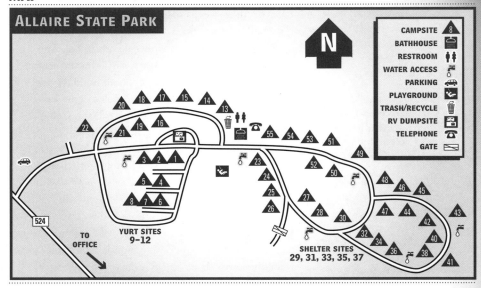

ALLAIRE STATE PARK

N

CAMPSITE	8
BATHHOUSE	
RESTROOM	
WATER ACCESS	
PARKING	
PLAYGROUND	
TRASH/RECYCLE	
RV DUMPSITE	
TELEPHONE	
GATE	

524

TO OFFICE

YURT SITES 9–12

SHELTER SITES 29, 31, 33, 35, 37

will link Trenton and the Atlantic Coast via a scenic greenway.

The Manasquan River winds through the park and is stocked seasonally with trout. Anglers have reportedly caught sea-run brown trout as large as four pounds within Allaire, which has three stocking points. Canoeing and kayaking the east-running river is also popular. Several boat rental agencies are nearby.

When James P. Allaire purchased Howell Works, he lobbied hard for better transportation connections between Monmouth County and New York City. He'd be pleased if he were alive today. His former company is not only a destination in and of itself, but is conveniently located at the nexus of two major highways, I-195 and the Garden State Parkway. But you wouldn't know it from within the campground. The roar of civilization is far away from the shaded sites.

GETTING THERE

From the Garden State Parkway, take Exit 98 and follow signs to Allaire State Park. From I-195, take Exit 31B to County Road 524 East.

BULL'S ISLAND RECREATION AREA

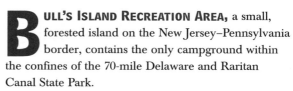

> *Choose from the walk-in riverfront or canal-facing sites and your only neighbor may be a duck.*

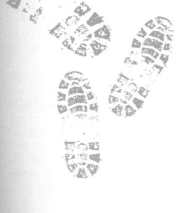

BULL'S ISLAND RECREATION AREA, a small, forested island on the New Jersey–Pennsylvania border, contains the only campground within the confines of the 70-mile Delaware and Raritan Canal State Park.

The park itself is linear, following the route of the D&R Canal and its feeder canal that parallels NJ 29 along the coast. Although it encompasses 70 miles, much of the park is no more than 25 yards wide. The D&R Canal was one of two canals that crossed New Jersey during the Industrial Revolution, carrying coal from Pennsylvania to New York and transporting goods in reverse. The Morris Canal connected New York Harbor and Phillipsburg, with mules pulling barges a distance of 102 miles over five days. Today that same trip, along I-78, takes a truck just over an hour. Most of the Morris Canal is paved over or has been used in the construction of streetcar or subway lines. The eastern terminus of the Morris Canal is beside Liberty State Park in Jersey City, alongside Liberty Harbor RV Park (tents allowed).

The fates were kinder to the D&R Canal than to the Morris Canal. The State of New Jersey adopted it as a water supply line, keeping it mostly intact. Locals realized that the towpath was ideal for cycling and hiking, and in 1974 the de facto recreation area became a state park.

Bull's Island is sandwiched between the Delaware River and the D&R feeder canal, making it inaccessible to cars except through the lockable front gate. A row of sites along the tip of the island is designated walk-in; these are accessible to foot traffic only. Choose from riverfront sites 64 through 69 or canal-facing sites 56 through 63 and your only neighbor may be a duck. But humans are not a problem—thick undergrowth gives campers the illusion of isolation on the bush

RATINGS

Beauty: ✿ ✿ ✿ ✿
Privacy: ✿ ✿ ✿
Spaciousness: ✿ ✿ ✿ ✿
Quiet: ✿ ✿ ✿
Security: ✿ ✿ ✿ ✿ ✿
Cleanliness: ✿ ✿ ✿

riverbank. The Weir Dam is to the left of site 69, making this an ideal location to sit and watch the Delaware swirl. A parking area is located just 50 to 100 yards away, with flushing toilets only a short distance beyond that. Those who need to keep their cars closer can book sites 53 through 55, which are less private but look right over the dam. Trailer owners should note that there are no hookups at Bull's Island.

Drive-in sites line six other loops, with varying degrees of shade and privacy. Sites 4 through 30 sit under the occasional maple or birch tree around a large, flat field. You won't find privacy barriers on the field, but there is light for sunseekers. These sites are ideal for multiple family groups.

A boat launch is located just beyond the visitor center, next to the footbridge to Pennsylvania. Bring or rent a canoe and drift along the Delaware. Private canoe rental agencies are located nearby, as are tubing companies. Tubing out of Frenchtown or Stockton may bring you into contact with a local legend—The Hot Dog Man—who plies his trade in the middle of the Delaware. Wet money is acceptable. Canoes, kayaks, and small boats (electric motors) are allowed on the canal. Boaters must carry their boats over the locks.

Horses are not allowed along the feeder canal but are permitted on the main canal towpath. The trail along the feeder canal is popular with hikers and cyclists. You can rent bikes in nearby Stockton, which is also home to nineteenth-century Prallsville Mills. The site contains a sawmill, gristmill, and linseed oil mill. Cycling farther south will take you to Washington Crossing State Park, the site of the Continental Army's landing in 1776, before their historic march to Trenton. This 1,773-acre park contains animals, multiuse trails, and historic buildings, but its campground is for groups only.

Fishing is popular at Bull's Island and throughout the D&R Canal State Park, although signs in the region warn of the possibility of high mercury levels in local fish. Those lucky enough to be staying along the water can fish directly from campsites. Fishing on the canal side may produce catfish, eel, rock bass, and trout. The Delaware River side is more likely to be home to

KEY INFORMATION

ADDRESS:	Delaware & Raritan Canal State Park Bull's Island Recreation Area 2185 Daniel Bray Highway Stockton, NJ 08559
OPERATED BY:	State Park Service
INFORMATION:	(609) 397-2949
WEB SITE:	www.dandrcanal.com
OPEN:	April–October
SITES:	69
EACH SITE HAS:	Picnic table, fire ring
ASSIGNMENT:	In advance or choose from available sites
REGISTRATION:	On arrival or reserve minimum 2 nights
FACILITIES:	Water, flush toilets, showers
PARKING:	At site, 2-vehicle limit
FEE:	$15
ELEVATION:	80 feet
RESTRICTIONS:	Pets: Prohibited Fires: In fire rings only Alcohol: Prohibited Vehicles: No limit; no hookups Other: Quiet hours 10 p.m.–6 a.m.; all guests must obtain permit from office; 14-night, 6-person, and 2-tent limit; no group camping.

MAP

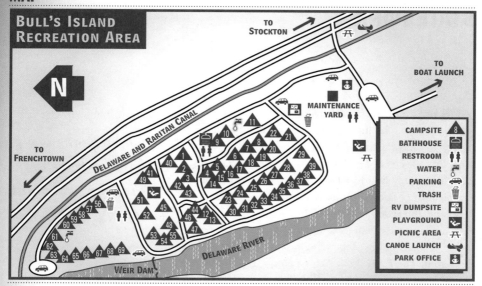

BULL'S ISLAND RECREATION AREA

TO STOCKTON

TO BOAT LAUNCH

N

TO FRENCHTOWN

DELAWARE AND RARITAN CANAL

MAINTENANCE YARD

DELAWARE RIVER

WEIR DAM

CAMPSITE	8
BATHHOUSE	
RESTROOM	
WATER	
PARKING	
TRASH	
RV DUMPSITE	
PLAYGROUND	
PICNIC AREA	
CANOE LAUNCH	
PARK OFFICE	

GETTING THERE

From I-287, take Exit 17 and go south on US 202 for 26 miles. Exit onto NJ 29 North just before the toll bridge at the Delaware River. Drive north 6 miles to the park entrance on the left.

smallmouth bass, pickerel, sunfish, suckers, carp, and shad in addition to catfish and rock bass. Trout is stocked in some parts of the canal.

Bull's Island Natural Area, with its mixture of lowland floodplain forest, natural beauty, river and towpath access, and security, is one of the top public campgrounds in New Jersey. Reserve in advance during the summer and on weekends.

CHEESEQUAKE STATE PARK

Matawan

CHEESEQUAKE BEARS THE RESPONSIBILITY of being the most urban state park in the densest, most urbanized state in the country. A mere 36 miles from Manhattan, its wooded and marsh 1,292 acres play host to swimmers, anglers, hikers, bikers, picnickers, sports enthusiasts, small mammals, deer, and 186 species of birds. The Garden State Parkway, a congested coastal toll highway that can be scenic or aggravating (depending on traffic), runs right through it. The PNC Bank Arts Center, a 17,500-seat amphitheater that features multimillion-dollar live concerts, is only 8 miles away.

But its disadvantages are also advantages: Travelers who want to be near New York happily set up tents here; concert-goers enjoy Cheesequake for its access to the arts center; and its proximity to the Garden State Parkway makes Cheesequake desirable for the budget-conscious who want to be near Jersey's northern beaches.

Even without the local attractions, Cheesequake is a destination in its own right. Its ecosystem is diverse, as it lies in the transitional zone between northern and southern Jersey. Cheesequake features salt and freshwater marshes as well as pine barrens and a northeastern hardwood forest.

The campground is located on the southeastern edge of the park, in a relatively unspoiled area. Most of the trails and recreational facilities are located across the Garden State Parkway. The Stump Creek area north of the campground is completely undeveloped.

The 53 quiet campsites are impeccably maintained. The forest canopy shades all sites, and the vegetation between sites makes the spacious sites seem even more private. Firewood is sometimes supplied with each site. Two dead-end spurs house the quietest, most secluded sites. Unfortunately, they are farthest from the

> *Cheesequake is a great base for traveling campers who want to tour New York City.*

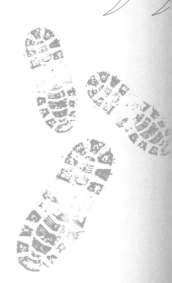

RATINGS

Beauty: ☆ ☆ ☆
Privacy: ☆ ☆ ☆
Spaciousness: ☆ ☆ ☆ ☆
Quiet: ☆ ☆ ☆
Security: ☆ ☆ ☆
Cleanliness: ☆ ☆ ☆ ☆

KEY INFORMATION

ADDRESS:	Cheesequake State Park 300 Gordon Road Matawan, NJ 07747
OPERATED BY:	State Park Service
INFORMATION:	(732) 566-2161
WEB SITE:	www.njparksand forests.org
OPEN:	April–October
SITES:	53
EACH SITE HAS:	Picnic table, fire ring
ASSIGNMENT:	On arrival; requests considered but not guaranteed
REGISTRATION:	On arrival or reserve minimum 2 nights
FACILITIES:	Water, flush toilets, showers
PARKING:	At site, maximum 2 vehicles
FEE:	$15
ELEVATION:	10 feet
RESTRICTIONS:	Pets: Prohibited Fires: In fire rings only Alcohol: Prohibited Vehicles: 11-foot height limit Other: No cutting of live trees; quiet hours 10 p.m.–6 a.m.; 14-night, 6-person, and 2-tent limit; no refunds due to biting insects

single bathhouse and closest to Laurence Harbor Parkway, with its cars and new housing development. A tall fence and some understory separate the campground from the road.

The entrance fee comes with a disclaimer: "There will be no entrance fee refund due to the seasonal insect problem." Parts of Cheesequake are located on a salt marsh, complete with resident mosquitoes, biting flies, and midges. The campground is not in the salt marsh, but be prepared to deal with insects as you use some of the recreational facilities.

Sandy Hook, a 1,665-acre barrier beach peninsula, is located 15 minutes away via Exit 117 of the Garden State Parkway. Part of the Gateway National Recreation Area, it features a fort, exhibits, fishing, hiking, and the oldest operating lighthouse in the country. Swimming and ocean sports are popular at Sandy Hook, but camping is only open to organized groups.

Those with a fear of sharks and an overactive imagination may prefer to swim in six-acre Hooks Creek Lake at Cheesequake. Forty-foot-wide tidal Matawan Creek—right where it meets the Garden State Parkway at milepost 119.4—was the unlikely site of three of the five shark attacks in 1916 later made famous in *Jaws*. Fortunately, no sharks have been seen in Matawan in nine decades, and Matawan Creek does not connect with landlocked Hooks Creek Lake.

Anglers catch trout, largemouth bass, catfish, and sunfish in the lake. Cheesequake is also renowned for its crabbing, which can be done from the crabbing bridge. Access is from the lake parking lot.

Four of Cheesequake's five trails are for hiking only, while the remaining 3.5-mile single-track trail is also open to cyclists. Trails are classified as easy to moderate and have some inclines. The longest hiking trail is the Green Trail, a 3.5-mile loop that passes by examples of the various ecosystems that make up Cheesequake State Park. First, you'll walk by a salt marsh before going through a hardwood forest. You'll pass under pitch pines before continuing on to a freshwater swamp and a white cedar swamp. Finally, the trail passes 150-year-old white pines before ending back at the parking area.

MAP

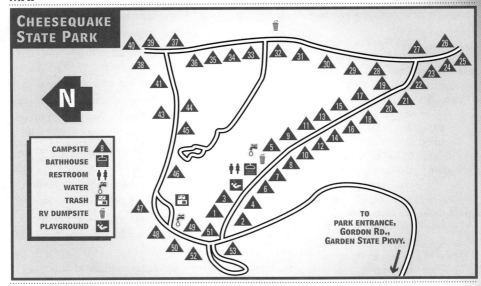

CHEESEQUAKE STATE PARK

N

CAMPSITE	8
BATHHOUSE	
RESTROOM	
WATER	
TRASH	
RV DUMPSITE	
PLAYGROUND	

TO
PARK ENTRANCE,
GORDON RD.,
GARDEN STATE PKWY.

Cheesequake is a great base for traveling campers who want to tour New York City. Park your car in Matawan at the train station and catch one of the frequent New Jersey Transit commuter trains to New York's Penn Station.

The Raritan Bay area was originally inhabited by the Lenni Lenape Native Americans. They called the area "land which has been declared," or "chis-kahki." We call it "Cheesequake," which rhymes with cheesecake. Inquiring about the availability of cheesecake at Cheesequake will only get you a glare, much as one gets from a native New Jerseyan after delivering the tired old line, "You're from Jersey? What exit?" But you will find shaded campsites, plenty of wildlife, and many recreational opportunities in Cheesequake State Park.

GETTING THERE

From the Garden State Parkway, take Exit 120. Drive straight for 0.4 miles, following signs for Cheesequake State Park. Bear right on Laurence Habor Morristown Road/Matawan Road for 0.2 miles. Turn right onto Morristown Road for 0.3 miles. Go right at Gordon Road to the park entrance.

DELAWARE RIVER FAMILY CAMPGROUND

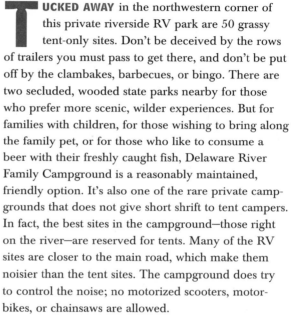

> *The river is the star attraction here, with boating, tubing, and fishing from its banks.*

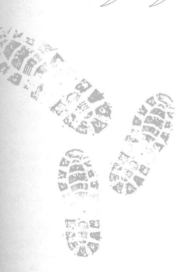

TUCKED AWAY in the northwestern corner of this private riverside RV park are 50 grassy tent-only sites. Don't be deceived by the rows of trailers you must pass to get there, and don't be put off by the clambakes, barbecues, or bingo. There are two secluded, wooded state parks nearby for those who prefer more scenic, wilder experiences. But for families with children, for those wishing to bring along the family pet, or for those who like to consume a beer with their freshly caught fish, Delaware River Family Campground is a reasonably maintained, friendly option. It's also one of the rare private campgrounds that does not give short shrift to tent campers. In fact, the best sites in the campground—those right on the river—are reserved for tents. Many of the RV sites are closer to the main road, which make them noisier than the tent sites. The campground does try to control the noise; no motorized scooters, motorbikes, or chainsaws are allowed.

The Delaware River is the star attraction here, and the camp offers rafting, canoeing, tubing, and kayaking in addition to allowing fishing from its banks. You can launch boats from the campground along with sit-down Jet Skis. Stand-up Jet Skis are not permitted on the Delaware. Swimming is allowed in the pool only and is not permitted on the beach or near the boat launch area.

Eight-mile rafting, canoeing, and kayaking trips are offered, with shuttle transportation included. Tubing trips are 4 miles long. Trips leave on the hour from 9 a.m. to 3 p.m. daily. Shuttles drop off tubers upstream, and the current brings them back. Canoes and motorized boats can also be rented for daily use. Fishing is not allowed from rafts, and life vests must always be worn. There is a three-beer-per-adult limit on the river, and U.S. park rangers have been known to enforce it.

RATINGS

Beauty: ✿ ✿
Privacy: ✿ ✿
Spaciousness: ✿ ✿ ✿
Quiet: ✿ ✿
Security: ✿ ✿ ✿
Cleanliness: ✿ ✿ ✿

Unlike at New Jersey state parks, pets are allowed at Delaware Family Campground. But there is a host of rules and regulations regarding our canine friends. Dogs must be leashed and attended, and all waste must be cleaned up immediately. Barking dogs are not tolerated, and pet owners must pay an additional $1 per night for each pet. No pit bulls, dobermans, chow-chows, rottweilers, wolf hybrids, or mixes of any of these will be allowed into the campground. All dogs must be up to date on their rabies vaccines.

The experience of camping in a private campground is distinctly different from that of setting up a tent in a pristine, secluded wilderness. But there are benefits to camping in an organized environment, particularly for those looking to entertain children. Delaware Family Campground offers a safe environment for kids to ride bicycles (helmets required) or swim in the pool. There is a playground, miniature golf course, basketball court, game room, and sand volleyball court. Mini carnivals are occasionally offered, along with clowns, magicians, and Christmas in July. Scavenger hunts, crafts, ice cream socials, and movie nights round out the possible offerings. Adult activities include workshops offered in ceramics, crafts, and golf.

Delaware Family Campground is centrally located for those wishing to make the climb up Mount Tammany at the Delaware Water Gap. Tear the kids away from tubing and swimming long enough to drive up to the Dunnfield parking area, near the Delaware Water Gap information center off I-80. Hike along the Red Dot Trail (Mount Tammany Trail) for 1.5 miles, rising 1,250 feet to the summit. The walk is rocky and moderately strenuous. You'll see dramatic views of the Gap and of Mount Minsi in Pennsylvania before hiking back down along the Blue Dot Trail.

Delaware Family Campground comes with its own "distinctly Delaware" rules. Firewood must be purchased on site. Wristbands must be worn at all times, identifying campers as paying members of the community; gate cards must be rented or tokens purchased to get in and out of the campground. Only white T-shirts are allowed to be worn over bathing

KEY INFORMATION

ADDRESS: Delaware River Family Campground P.O. Box 142 100 US 46 Delaware, NJ 07833

OPERATED BY: Private

INFORMATION: (908) 475-1006

WEB SITE: www.drfcnj.com

OPEN: Year-round

SITES: 50

EACH SITE HAS: Picnic table, fire ring

ASSIGNMENT: On arrival

REGISTRATION: On arrival or reserve minimum 2 nights

FACILITIES: Water, flush toilets, showers, laundry room, pay phones

PARKING: 1-car limit per site; additional parking at lot

FEE: Adult, $15; child, $5; per pet, $1; $3 per additional adult, $1 per additional child

ELEVATION: 300 feet

RESTRICTIONS: Pets: Must be on leash and attended; clean up after dogs; no pets on beach Fires: In fire rings only; must be out by midnight; must buy firewood on site Alcohol: 21 or older Vehicles: No limit Other: Quiet hours 11 p.m.–7 a.m.; no swimming in river; no firearms; licensed fishing only; no motorbikes; children on bikes must wear helmets

MAP

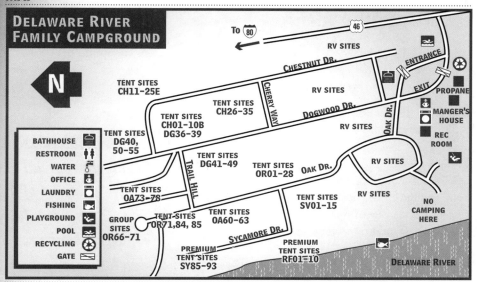

DELAWARE RIVER FAMILY CAMPGROUND

To 80 ←

46

RV SITES

CHESTNUT DR.

ENTRANCE

EXIT

PROPANE

TENT SITES
CH11-25E

TENT SITES
CH26-35

RV SITES

DOGWOOD DR.

MANGER'S
HOUSE

CHERRY WAY

TENT SITES
CH01-10B
DG36-39

RV SITES

OAK DR.

REC
ROOM

BATHHOUSE
RESTROOM
WATER
OFFICE
LAUNDRY
FISHING
PLAYGROUND
POOL
RECYCLING
GATE

TENT SITES
DG40,
50-55

TENT SITES
DG41-49

TENT SITES
OR01-28

OAK DR.

RV SITES

TRAIL HILL

TENT SITES
OA73-78

TENT SITES
SV01-15

RV SITES

NO
CAMPING
HERE

GROUP
SITES
OR66-71

TENT SITES
OR71,84, 85

TENT SITES
OA60-63

SYCAMORE DR.

PREMIUM
TENT SITES
SY85-93

PREMIUM
TENT SITES
RF01-10

DELAWARE RIVER

N

GETTING THERE

From I-80, take Exit 4B to US 46 East. The campground is 3 miles on the right.

suits in the pool. And you must leave your chainsaws and pit bulls at home, even if they seem like part of the family. But when it comes to pets and alcohol, the park allows for more relaxed camping than state parks.

ROUND VALLEY
RECREATION AREA

Lebanon

T HE **85 CAMPSITES** on the eastern shore of Round Valley Reservoir are among the most rustic developed sites in New Jersey. Officially termed "wilderness campsites," they are totally inaccessible by road. Sites spread out along 3.5 miles of lakefront, and the closest site to the parking area is a 3-mile hike away on a rugged trail.

Campers must carry in all gear and must carry out all garbage. Firewood may be gathered from the ground but cannot be cut from trees. Remember that New Jersey has an abundance of black bears, and you will have no car in which to lock your food. Bring along a bear-proof container and keep it away from your tent and out of reach. Do not put food residue into your campfire. Remember that feeding a bear teaches it to associate humans with food. See the Introduction for more information on how to camp safely in bear country.

The farthest campsites are 6 miles from the South Parking Lot. The sites are on a gravel path that runs parallel to Cushetunk Trail. Plenty of fresh water is available along the path. In addition to hiking in, campers can also travel to sites by boat or mountain bike.

Visitors can launch boats from the divers and campers boat ramp near the South Parking Lot. Only sailboats, canoes, or motorboats up to 10 horsepower are permitted. Life vests are required in vessels under 14 feet long. Sites 10, 13, 16, 22, 23, 26, 38, 40, 47, 48, 72, and group site 7 have good boat access and are close to the reservoir's edge. Watch for high winds; when wind speeds hit 20 mph, warning lights flash and boaters must immediately pull into shore. Boating campers would then have to wait or hike out of the campground. Do not ignore these warnings: Round Valley is known for strong winds that can be deadly.

> *These wilderness campsites spread out over 3.5 miles of lakefront and are totally inaccessible by road.*

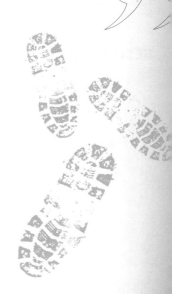

RATINGS

Beauty: ✿ ✿ ✿ ✿
Privacy: ✿ ✿ ✿ ✿
Spaciousness: ✿ ✿ ✿
Quiet: ✿ ✿ ✿ ✿ ✿
Security: ✿ ✿ ✿
Cleanliness: ✿ ✿ ✿

ADDRESS: Round Valley
Recreation Area
1220 Lebanon-
Stanton Road
Lebanon, NJ 08833

OPERATED BY: State Park Service

INFORMATION: (908) 236-6355

WEB SITE: www.njparksand
forests.org

OPEN: April–October

SITES: 85

EACH SITE HAS: Fire ring

ASSIGNMENT: First come, first
served

REGISTRATION: On arrival or
reserve minimum 2
nights

FACILITIES: Water, vault toilets,
pay phone

PARKING: At south parking lot;
3 miles to campsites

FEE: $12

ELEVATION: 400 feet

RESTRICTIONS: Pets: Prohibited
Fires: In fire rings
only
Alcohol: Prohibited
Vehicles: No limit;
no hookups
Other: Quiet hours
10 p.m.–6 a.m.; all
guests must obtain
permit from office;
14-night, 6-person,
and 2-tent limit; no
group camping; sites
must be vacated by
noon

Arrive early if you want to camp at Round Valley Recreation Area. Because of the long haul to the campground, no one is allowed to check in later than 4:30 p.m. (3:30 p.m. in October).

At 180 feet deep, man-made Round Valley Reservoir is New Jersey's deepest and second-largest lake. It is an ideal spot for those learning or practicing their open-water scuba skills. The diving area, a protected cove near the divers and campers boat ramp, is a maximum of 60 feet deep. Divers enter the water from the beach, and there is an underwater training platform in the cove. Diving groups are required to display the scuba flag while underwater and must check in and out at the Ranger Station. Certification and presentation of safety equipment are required to obtain a permit. Call ahead for details.

Snorkeling is allowed off the camping area by permit, provided all safety equipment has been presented and approved by rangers at the park entrance. If hiking in, remember you'll be carrying your mask, fins, and life vest in addition to camping gear and food. There is no boat rental concession at Round Valley, so getting a kayak or canoe to access the campsite will require some creative planning and forethought.

Round Valley Recreation Area is considered one of New Jersey's most challenging mountain biking spots. Bikers and hikers (and the occasional horse) share the rocky Cushetunk Trail for the first 3 miles, until the trail splits. Campers take the left fork down to the shore through 3 miles of carefully spaced campsites. The right fork goes up a ridge and continues for another 3 miles. Most bikers go right, testing their mettle on a challenging aerobic workout. They then return via the campground trail. Mountain biking at Round Valley consists of hard, sustained uphills, technical descents, and many rocks. It is not for beginners.

Swimming is not allowed off the camping area but is allowed at the day-use area when lifeguards are on duty. The day-use area is near the parking lot, 3 miles from the nearest campsites. The beach complex contains changing rooms, restrooms, showers, and concessionaires. No grilling is allowed on the beach, but three nearby picnic areas feature grills.

MAP

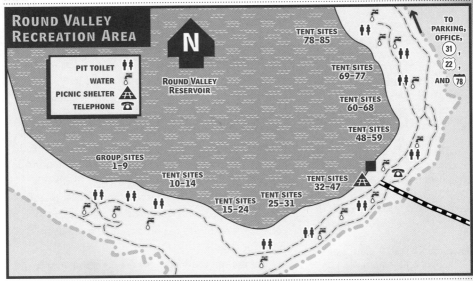

Anglers must follow special fishing regulations at Round Valley Reservoir, as it is one of New Jersey's two trophy trout lakes (Merrill Creek Reservoir is the other). Some of the largest trout in the state have been caught at Round Valley. Large bass and bluegill are also found there, and some anglers call Round Valley the "valley of the giants." Fishing is not allowed near the swimming area.

Between fishing, biking, and diving, there's no shortage of things to do at Round Valley. But there is a shortage of parking spaces, so get there early on summer weekends.

GETTING THERE

From I-78, take Exit 18 to US 22 East. Follow signs to the park.

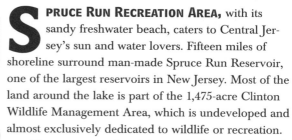

SPRUCE RUN
RECREATION AREA

> *Spruce Run Reservoir is renowned for its beach and excellent fishing opportunities.*

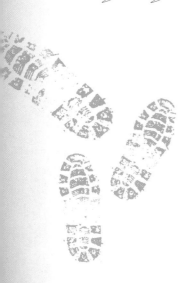

SPRUCE RUN RECREATION AREA, with its sandy freshwater beach, caters to Central Jersey's sun and water lovers. Fifteen miles of shoreline surround man-made Spruce Run Reservoir, one of the largest reservoirs in New Jersey. Most of the land around the lake is part of the 1,475-acre Clinton Wildlife Management Area, which is undeveloped and almost exclusively dedicated to wildlife or recreation.

The campground and day-use facilities are located on two peninsulas that jut into the water from the northern side of the lake. The campground lies at the tip of the larger peninsula and consists of three loops set around a large, grassy field. No electrical or water hookups are available, but there is a dump station. The spacious, open sites are used most frequently by multi-family groups who do not desire privacy barriers between sites. A few sites are shaded, but the real appeal is in the waterfront real estate. Sites along the outer rim of the campground sit directly on the 1,290-acre lake.

Spruce Run's campground may be lacking in shaded areas, but it does not lack conveniences. Both bathhouses contain showers, and the lakeside bath also has a dishwashing station. Additionally, the bathhouse by the swimming beach contains showers as well as changing areas, restrooms, a first-aid room, and concessions.

The beach is open for swimming Memorial Day weekend through Labor Day, when lifeguards are on duty. There is a playground as well as open fields for setting up ball games. Grilling is not allowed on the beach, but there are charcoal grills at the picnic areas. Visitors can bring their own grills to the picnic areas but not to the beach.

Swimmers are only allowed to enter the water from the beach, and not from campsites or boats. The reservoir is famed for its favorable sailing winds, and

RATINGS

Beauty: ☆ ☆ ☆ ☆
Privacy: ☆ ☆
Spaciousness: ☆ ☆ ☆
Quiet: ☆ ☆ ☆
Security: ☆ ☆ ☆
Cleanliness: ☆ ☆ ☆ ☆

several sailing events occur at the recreation area. Canoeing, kayaking, and motorized boating (less than 10 horsepower only) is popular. Boating is allowed 24 hours a day. A wind warning light flashes when wind speeds are too fast to cruise, reminding boaters to get to shore immediately.

Spruce Run Reservoir, along with its tributaries, is renowned for its excellent fishing opportunities. Both boat fishing and shoreline fishing are permitted. Thirty species of fish call the region home, with various types of trout, bass, catfish, and crappie stocked along with northern pike and tiger muskies. A drawdown has diminished aquatic vegetation, which in turn affected the populations of bass and northern pike, but other species are thriving. For anglers wishing to test their skills at Spruce Run, the New Jersey Division of Fish and Wildlife puts out a free digest that includes informative articles as well as rules and regulations. Pick one up at the visitor center.

Cyclists and runners use the park roadways and grounds, but the only major hiking trail at Spruce Run is a 0.9-mile portion of the Highlands Trail. The bistate trail will eventually connect New Jersey's Delaware River and the Hudson River in New York. The trail extends 126 miles north, but the southern terminus, as of the writing of this book, is 1.5 miles away from Spruce Run Recreation Area in Clinton Wildlife Management Area. While wandering the trail, keep an eye open for birds. Spruce Run is home to dozens of species. A birding checklist complete with visual profiles is available at the visitor center.

In addition to being sought after by picnickers, hikers, anglers, swimmers, boaters, and campers, these Hunterdon County hills are popular with deer, rabbits, ducks, turkeys, and small mammals. Public hunting is allowed in parts of the Clinton Wildlife Management Area during specific periods between September and January, while Spruce Run Recreation Area allows only seasonal waterfowl hunting. Waterfowl hunters are not allowed near the day-use or camping areas. Permits must be obtained for all hunting in New Jersey. Check the New Jersey Fish and Wildlife Digest,

KEY INFORMATION

ADDRESS:	Spruce Run Recreation Area 1 Van Syckel's Road Clinton, NJ 08809
OPERATED BY:	State Park Service
INFORMATION:	(908) 638-8572
WEB SITE:	www.njparksand forests.org
OPEN:	April–October
SITES:	70
EACH SITE HAS:	Picnic table, grill, lantern posts
ASSIGNMENT:	First come, first served
REGISTRATION:	On arrival or reserve minimum 2 nights
FACILITIES:	Water, flush toilets, showers
PARKING:	At site, 2-vehicle limit
FEE:	$15
ELEVATION:	300 feet
RESTRICTIONS:	**Pets:** Prohibited **Fires:** In grills only **Alcohol:** Prohibited **Vehicles:** No limit **Other:** Quiet hours 10 p.m.–6 a.m.; 14-night, 6-person, 2-tent limit

MAP

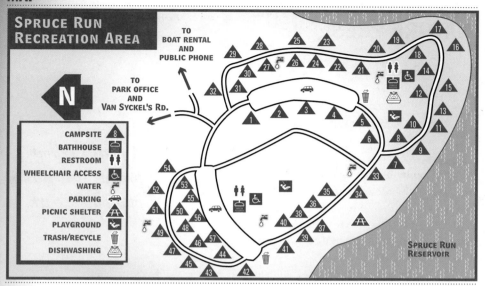

SPRUCE RUN RECREATION AREA

TO BOAT RENTAL AND PUBLIC PHONE

TO PARK OFFICE AND VAN SYCKEL'S RD.

N

CAMPSITE
BATHHOUSE
RESTROOM
WHEELCHAIR ACCESS
WATER
PARKING
PICNIC SHELTER
PLAYGROUND
TRASH/RECYCLE
DISHWASHING

SPRUCE RUN RESERVOIR

GETTING THERE

From I-78, take Exit 17. Follow NJ 31 North to the third traffic light. Turn left onto Van Syckel's Road. Drive 1.5 miles to the park entrance on the left.

available at the Spruce Run Visitor Center, for details as hunting seasons change yearly.

Consider a day trip to nearby Clinton, where you can stroll past two historic mills built in the 1700s. The Raritan River flows through town, and the mills flank it where it dips into a wide waterfall. The stone mill is currently used as an art museum, and the red mill houses a Hunterdon County history museum along with community and school programs. Many of Clinton's original buildings burned down in 1891, but the townspeople immediately began to rebuild. Today the historic center is filled with boutiques and specialty shops.

Special events occur regularly on the Spruce Run grounds, so keep your eyes open for walk-a-thons, triathlons, weddings, watershed cleanup days, and sailing events. But the reservoir, with its beach and fishing opportunities, is worth a visit any time.

TEETERTOWN RAVINE NATURE PRESERVE

LOCAL FAMILIES WILL LOVE these serene wilderness sites tucked away in this densely wooded haven in Hunterdon County, near the Morris County border. Opened in June of 2003, the five sites of the Mountain Farm section of Teetertown Ravine Nature Preserve are spread out along a forest trail. It's a half-mile hike from the parking lot, but campers are rewarded with their own private, tree-lined sanctuaries.

No shortcuts to the sites exist, and campers must carry in all supplies, including water. There's a faucet at the parking area, and those with excess equipment can borrow garden carts from the staff. The inconvenience of the sites is by design, not by accident. The sites are geared toward nature lovers and those truly seeking a backcountry experience. Campers hike between 0.5 to 0.75 miles and pass by small mammals, birds, rock outcroppings, and a pond before they get to the sites.

Hikers are rewarded for their efforts when they reach some of the nicest, newest campsites in New Jersey. Sites are spread out across two groups and are isolated from other sites. Sites within groupings are connected by paths. They are distant enough to ensure privacy but close enough to allow multiple sites to be used with a single reservation. Each site has a fireside bench in addition to the standard picnic table and fire ring. Adjustable cooking surfaces sit above the fire rings, and each site accommodates two tents. Two portable toilets are a nod to convenience in this rustic area, as are the mulch tent pads, ground to a fine powdery base for sleeping comfort.

Hunterdon County's first public camping facility is a perfect example of private stewardship of public parks. The grounds, which are still being procured, were acquired through the cooperation of multiple

> *A perfect example of private stewardship of a public park.*

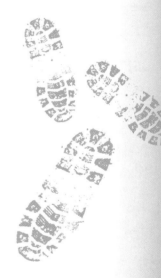

RATINGS

Beauty: ✿ ✿ ✿ ✿ ✿
Privacy: ✿ ✿ ✿ ✿ ✿
Spaciousness: ✿ ✿ ✿ ✿
Quiet: ✿ ✿ ✿ ✿ ✿
Security: ✿ ✿ ✿
Cleanliness: ✿ ✿ ✿ ✿ ✿

KEY INFORMATION

ADDRESS: Teetertown Ravine Natural Area
30 Pleasant Grove Road
Lebanon Township, NJ 07865

OPERATED BY: Hunterdon County Park System

INFORMATION: (908) 782-1158

WEB SITE: www.co.hunterdon.nj.us

OPEN: Year-round conditions permitting; weekends only

SITES: 5

EACH SITE HAS: Picnic table, fire ring, bench, firewood

ASSIGNMENT: First come, first served; requests honored

REGISTRATION: In advance in person or download Web site form

FACILITIES: Portable toilets, water at parking area

PARKING: At central lot; hike to sites

FEE: $15; county residents, $10

ELEVATION: 1,000 feet

RESTRICTIONS: Pets: On leash; must sleep in occupied tent; prohibited in ponds and grasslands
Fires: In fire rings with permit; use firewood supplied
Alcohol: Prohibited
Vehicles: None
Other: 6-person, 2-tent limit per site; collecting downed wood prohibited

public organizations, but the labor was nearly all volunteer. Almost all building materials were recycled from other projects. Materials for the group camping parking lot and the single-lane road that winds through the picnic area, for example, were recycled from remnants of a nearby country road, which was repaved with new materials.

Boy Scout Eagle Projects, Mountain Farm Campmaster Corps, Student Conservation Association, students and faculty of the Educational Service Commission at Mountain Farm, park staff, and individual volunteers all worked together to identify and build the camping area, picnic area, and trails. Volunteers cleared the land, dug out hundreds of boulders, framed sections, restored old picnic tables, and graded sites. They surrounded each concrete fireplace base with a two-foot bed of quarry millings. Volunteers even staff the visitor center on weekends.

Teetertown Ravine Nature Preserve, accessed from the camping area via a trail and steep footpath, is a geologist's paradise. Dense rock called "Diabase" was quarried from the area between 1896 and 1923. Today these rocks, along with a softer type called "Gneiss," adorn the green ravine. The quiet gorge is bisected by a paved road and bubbling stream. Rock climbing is illegal and strictly prohibited.

When the ravine was a quarry, the rocks were carried out on a purpose-built 1.3-mile-long railroad that went from the ravine to the main Central Railroad line. The small line closed with the quarry, and the last train ran on the Central route in 1976. Today the main line has been transformed into the Columbia Trail, a 7-mile hiking and biking trail that goes all the way to High Bridge, the weekday terminus of New Jersey Transit's Raritan Valley line.

Fishing is popular in the small ponds, which have healthy populations of bass and sunfish. Native trout can be found in Hollow Brook. Pond fishing is catch-and-release only.

Sites are open on weekends only, with the earliest check-in allowed on Friday at 5 p.m. Confirm check-in times in advance so that staff or volunteers will be present. Campers must break camp by noon on Sunday but

MAP

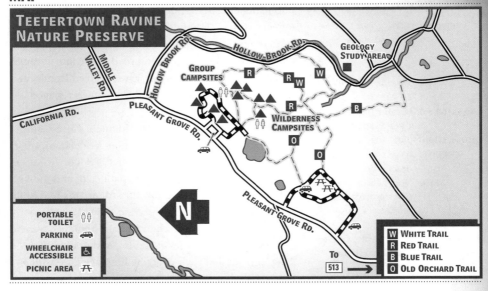

are free to use the trails, ponds, fields, and picnic tables of the preserve until closing time at the end of the day.

Firewood is included with the fee at Mountain Farm, and this is also part of the park's effort to maintain the natural habitat. Small mammals live on the forest floor and use the brush as cover. Don't use the brush and fallen limbs for your fire; use the firewood provided.

Sites must be reserved in advance. You can also use the form on the Hunterdon County Parks and Recreation Department Web site. Walk-ins are not accepted. Both the Mountain Farm section and Teetertown Ravine cannot be found on online map services by using Lebanon Township as a destination. The nearest post office is in Port Murray, so type in 30 Pleasant Grove Road, Port Murray, New Jersey, when searching for directions.

The usual warnings about bears and ticks apply. See the Introduction for more information on how to camp safely in bear country. Use sensible precautions to make your stay at New Jersey's newest sites an enjoyable one.

GETTING THERE

From I-78, take Exit 17 and drive north on NJ 31 for 1.7 miles. Turn right onto County Road 513 and proceed north through High Bridge. After 6.5 miles, turn left onto Sliker Road. Drive 1.5 miles. Turn right onto Pleasant Grove Road. The entrance to the Mountain Farm section of Teetertown Ravine Natural Area is on the right. Directions from other roads are on the Web site.

TRIPLE BROOK CAMPING RESORT

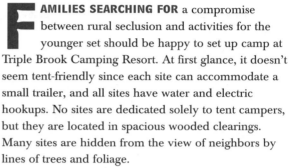

> *Unexpectedly wooded and scenic, Triple Brook is the only campground in New Jersey to feature 'cow plop bingo.'*

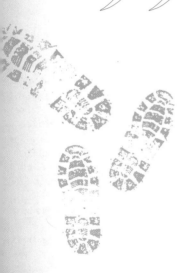

FAMILIES SEARCHING FOR a compromise between rural seclusion and activities for the younger set should be happy to set up camp at Triple Brook Camping Resort. At first glance, it doesn't seem tent-friendly since each site can accommodate a small trailer, and all sites have water and electric hookups. No sites are dedicated solely to tent campers, but they are located in spacious wooded clearings. Many sites are hidden from the view of neighbors by lines of trees and foliage.

Don't be put off by the sight of dozens of RVs lined up around a sunny field when you first enter the campground. Instead, drive straight down the main road until it ends. To the right is a line of open sites under a line of trees. These sites are popular with groups or multifamily parties. To the left are several wooded loops. Follow the one-way loop directly to the left as sites become increasingly more private. Finally, as you veer back toward the main road, you'll pass by sites as secluded as any you'll find in New Jersey's lovely public campgrounds. Some sites even sit beside a small creek.

Triple Brook does not allow pets, but it does supply its own. The 250-acre campground is a working farm, and visitors are welcome to visit the resident cows, chickens, and pigs. The farm grows crops, planting in spring and harvesting in autumn. Campers are welcome to observe and "experience" farm life. This applies to the more leisurely aspects of farm living, such as going on hayrides and petting horses, and not to being forced out of bed at five in the morning to milk rows of cows and goats.

Boating and fishing are allowed in the small lake, and boat rentals are available. All fishing is catch-and-release. The use of barbed hooks is prohibited. No glass containers are allowed by the lake. Frog-jumping

RATINGS

Beauty: ✿ ✿ ✿
Privacy: ✿ ✿
Spaciousness: ✿ ✿ ✿ ✿
Quiet: ✿ ✿ ✿
Security: ✿ ✿ ✿ ✿
Cleanliness: ✿ ✿ ✿ ✿

contests and earthworm races are held at the pond every Saturday during the summer.

Triple Brook also features a miniature golf course, swimming pool, small adults-only pool, adults-only spa, volleyball net, basketball court, horseshoe pit, and tennis court. A few cabins and rental RVs are available in addition to the many campsites. Plus, Triple Brook claims the distinction of being the only campground in New Jersey to feature "cow plop bingo."

Cow plop bingo is one of many games played on Bovine Weekend. Contestants choose a square in the pasture and must then wait for some time to see if their square receives the most manure deposits over the course of the afternoon. "Poo Sculpture" is another of the competitions. Although, it is, of course, much more highbrow than bingo. "It's a lot to doo with poo" is the weekend's slogan.

Brenda James and her family run Triple Brook. Many credit James with the folksy hospitality and event-planning spirit that keeps the campground unique. The family plans events just about every weekend, including the usual Easter egg hunts, movie nights, and ice cream socials, in addition to the more unique pots-and-pans parade, Christmas in July, and renowned teddy bear tea. Children are encouraged to bring their teddy bears to storytelling time; plenty of adults bring their teddy bears, too.

Triple Brook is centrally located near many of central Jersey's star attractions. Jenny Jump State Forest is a short drive away, with its hiking trails and Saturday night public access to the United Astronomy Clubs observatory. The Delaware Water Gap, with trails, canoeing, and fishing, is only 7 miles away. Lakota Wolf Preserve at Camp Taylor is nearby, and New York City is an hour's drive to the East. Other local attractions include amusement park Land of Make Believe, horse and pony stables, and the village of Hope. Originally a religious Moravian settlement, Hope is on the New Jersey and National Historic Registers.

Anglers can take an interesting day trip 7 miles away to the Pequest Trout Hatchery. The center is open daily, except on holidays, from 10 a.m. to 4 p.m.

KEY INFORMATION

ADDRESS: Triple Brook Camping Resort 58 Honey Run Road Hope, NJ 07825

OPERATED BY: Private

INFORMATION: (908) 459-4079

WEB SITE: www.triplebrook. com

OPEN: April–October

SITES: 100 appropriate for tents

EACH SITE HAS: Picnic table, fire ring

ASSIGNMENT: In advance or on arrival

REGISTRATION: On arrival or reserve minimum 2 nights

FACILITIES: Water, flush toilets, showers, pay phone laundry

PARKING: 1-car limit per wooded site; additional parking in lot

FEE: 2 people, $30; additional child, $5; additional adult, $1

ELEVATION: 600 feet

RESTRICTIONS: Pets: Prohibited
Fires: In fire rings only
Alcohol: Permitted at sites; prohibited in pool
Vehicles: No limit
Other: No strings of lights; no gathering or cutting firewood no electric bug zappers; 6-person limit in wooded areas; quiet hours 11 p.m.– 8 a.m.

MAP

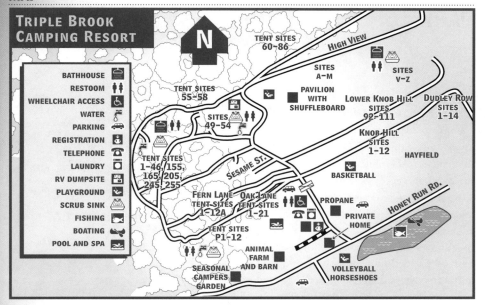

TRIPLE BROOK CAMPING RESORT

N

TENT SITES 60-86

HIGH VIEW

SITES A-M

SITES V-Z

TENT SITES 55-58

PAVILION WITH SHUFFLEBOARD

LOWER KNOB HILL SITES 92-111

DUDLEY ROW SITES 1-14

SITES 49-54

KNOB HILL SITES 1-12

HAYFIELD

TENT SITES 1-46, 155, 165, 205, 245, 255

SESAME ST.

BASKETBALL

FERN LANE TENT SITES 1-12A

OAK LANE TENT SITES 1-21

PROPANE

PRIVATE HOME

HONEY RUN RD.

TENT SITES P1-12

ANIMAL FARM AND BARN

VOLLEYBALL HORSESHOES

SEASONAL CAMPERS GARDEN

Legend:
- BATHHOUSE
- RESTOOM
- WHEELCHAIR ACCESS
- WATER
- PARKING
- REGISTRATION
- TELEPHONE
- LAUNDRY
- RV DUMPSITE
- PLAYGROUND
- SCRUB SINK
- FISHING
- BOATING
- POOL AND SPA

GETTING THERE

From I-80, take Exit 12 to County Road 521 south toward Hope. After 1 mile, turn right onto CR 609. After 3.5 miles, turn right onto Nightingale Road. Drive 1 mile and then turn right onto Honey Run Road. The campground entrance is a half mile on the left.

Visitors watch a video that demonstrates the trout-raising process and then can view the real thing.

Triple Brook, in the foothills of the Kittatinny Mountains, is not the right place for campers looking for a weekend of solitude and stargazing. But for families needing entertainment options along with their natural retreat, it offers a great balance between the outdoors and organized activities.

TURKEY SWAMP PARK

DESPITE ITS UNUSUAL NAME, this gem of a county park is not a swamp overrun with gobbling turkeys. The turkey in question was once the name of Adelphia, a nearby town. The park and surrounding Turkey Swamp Wildlife Management Area are located on sandy land just above the water table. Groundwater sometimes appears on the surface as small bogs.

Turkey Swamp's campsites are among the region's best: 64 wooded sites lie under a canopy of trees at the northern edge of the Pinelands, a protected unique ecosystem covering 1.1 million acres of land that includes swamps, farms, and forests. Although the overall campground is a compact crisscrossed loop, sites are spacious enough to accommodate large trailers. Privacy is assured by green undergrowth, pitch pines, and tall oak trees between sites. The bathhouse features hot showers, flushing toilets, and laundry facilities. Unfortunately, there is only one bathhouse for all 64 sites.

From the campground entrance, it is a short walk to the boathouse on the banks of the central 17-acre lake. Originally, the lake was man-made, but now it is sustained by natural springs that feed the lake. Visitors can rent paddleboats, rowboats, and canoes by the half hour; you must wear a life vest. Fishing for bass, catfish, and bluegill is popular from boats and from the shore. Swimming in the lake is prohibited, but campers may use the swimming pool at the Nomoco Activity Area on a limited basis when programs are not being conducted. Ice-skating on the lake is permissible when the water freezes in winter, although the campground is closed from December until March.

It is also possible to use Turkey Swamp as a base for canoeing or kayaking the Manasquan River. Boats rented in the park cannot be removed from the lake, but there are commercial rental agencies nearby.

> *Its proximity to natu[re], theme parks, and the beach should keep everyone in the family happy, even the dog.*

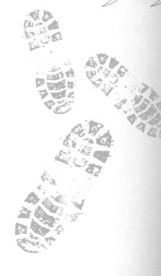

RATINGS

Beauty: ✫ ✫ ✫ ✫
Privacy: ✫ ✫ ✫
Spaciousness: ✫ ✫ ✫
Quiet: ✫ ✫ ✫
Security: ✫ ✫ ✫
Cleanliness: ✫ ✫ ✫ ✫

ADDRESS:	Turkey Swamp Park 66 Nomoco Road Freehold, NJ 07728
OPERATED BY:	Monmouth County Park System
INFORMATION:	(732) 462-7286
WEB SITE:	www.monmouth countyparks.com
OPEN:	March 15– November 30
SITES:	64; 14 for tents only
EACH SITE HAS:	Picnic table, fire ring, lantern post
ASSIGNMENT:	First come, first served
REGISTRATION:	On arrival or reserve minimum 2 nights
FACILITIES:	Water, flush toilets, showers, laundry, pay phones, vending machines
PARKING:	2-vehicle limit per site; overflow parking at entrance
FEE:	$27
ELEVATION:	130 feet
RESTRICTIONS:	Pets: Dogs must be on leash and attended Fires: Allowed in fire rings 7 a.m.–11 p.m. only Alcohol: Prohibited Vehicles: No limit Other: No collecting dead or live wood; quiet hours 10 p.m.– 8 a.m.

The 4 miles of trails in 1,180-acre Turkey Swamp Park are level. The mile-long fitness trail with its 20 exercise stations provides the only challenging option. Puddles of water occasionally bubble up through the trails. Trails are designated multiuse, although mountain bikers often scoff at the easy trails. Turkey Swamp's thorny trails will eventually be part of the statewide "Capital to the Coast" trail that will go from the Atlantic Ocean to Trenton, roughly paralleling I-195.

The adjacent state-managed Turkey Swamp Wildlife Management Area features an archery range that is run jointly by the Monmouth County Park System and the New Jersey Division of Fish, Game, and Wildlife. It is open to the public for training and practice. The Wildlife Management Area is open to deer hunting during varying autumn and winter weeks; behave sensibly during deer season.

In addition to being a recreational destination, Turkey Swamp makes a good base camp for family holidays. It is near Monmouth Battlefield State Park, site of one of the largest battles of the American Revolution and currently home to restored fences, lanes, and a farmhouse. It is supposedly the site of Molly Pitcher's Well. Molly Pitcher was known as the heroine of the Monmouth battle, but legend has overtaken fact and no one is certain what her actual role on the battlefield was. Arrive around June 28 to see the annual battle reenactment in which none other than General George Washington commands the Continental Army. He and his forces spent more time in New Jersey than in any other state, in part due to its key location between New York and Philadelphia.

For those looking for other types of fun, the Atlantic Ocean and Jersey shore are a short drive to the east, while the thrill-ride theme park Six Flags Great Adventure is an equally short drive to the west. Nearby Freehold is home to a horse raceway and the Old Tennent Presbyterian Church built in 1751. It is also the hometown of rock-and-roll icon Bruce Springsteen. Walking tours visit two of his former homes.

Those wishing to visit New York City on a day trip can take New Jersey Transit's North Jersey Coast

MAP

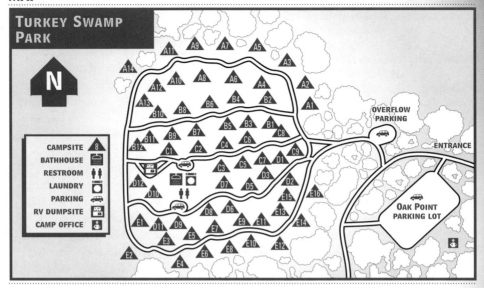

Line from Spring Lake or Belmar. Alternatively, commuter buses leave from Freehold. Inquire at the campground office for details.

Turkey Swamp campground is the only public campground in Central Jersey that allows campers to bring their dogs for overnight stays. It is unique among public campgrounds in its combination of natural forest, friendliness to dogs, and modern amenities. Its proximity to nature, theme parks, and the beach should keep everyone in the family happy, including the dog.

GETTING THERE

From I-195, take Exit 22. Turn north onto Jackson Mills Road and then left onto Georgia Road for 1.7 miles.

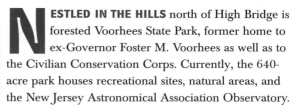

VOORHEES STATE PARK

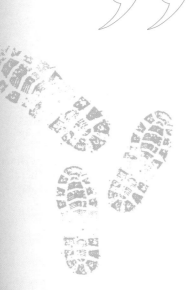

> *Many of the trails, trees, and structures at Voorhees were built by the CCC in the 1930s.*

NESTLED IN THE HILLS north of High Bridge is forested Voorhees State Park, former home to ex-Governor Foster M. Voorhees as well as to the Civilian Conservation Corps. Currently, the 640-acre park houses recreational sites, natural areas, and the New Jersey Astronomical Association Observatory.

The campground has no hookups, but this does not stop small RV owners from driving up the hill to the grassy sites. Tent campers may initially be dismayed by the sunny, open field and the trailers. Don't be fooled. Follow the small road as it disappears into the trees behind a "no RVs" sign. The sites beyond are shady, secluded, and green.

Three roads cross a triangle housing two dozen wooded alcoves. Continue to the far loop, on the north side of the field, to find the most private area. Sites 42 through 48 are small clearings carved out of wild vines and shrubs, set against a wilderness that seems ready to encroach on unaware campers. These sites are farther from the bathhouse but are ideal for those desiring solitude.

On the way to the campground, there is a scenic overlook. This viewpoint offers an expansive view of Hunterdon County and Round Valley Reservoir. Farther up Hill Acres Road is the Vista Trail, which leads to another overlook that faces Spruce Run Reservoir.

The parking lot by the Vista Trail is also next to the trailhead for the 1.5-mile Cross Park Trail, a pedestrian-only trail that connects the northern and southern parts of Voorhees. Cross Park Trail is part of the in-progress 150-mile Highlands Trail, which will connect the Delaware River with New York's Hudson River. Hikers can also try the 5 miles of trails at nearby Hacklebarney State Park. Voorhees' only other pedestrian-only trail is the 1-mile Parcourse circuit, a fitness route with 18 exercise stations. The remaining

RATINGS

Beauty: ✿ ✿ ✿ ✿
Privacy: ✿ ✿ ✿ ✿
Spaciousness: ✿ ✿ ✿
Quiet: ✿ ✿ ✿ ✿
Security: ✿ ✿ ✿
Cleanliness: ✿ ✿ ✿

five trails are designated multiuse, but most are too short for a satisfying bike ride. If you bring your bike, try combining Hill Acres Trail with the Brookside-Tanglewood loop. Swimming is not permitted in Willoughby Brook or in Voorhees' tiny ponds. Campers are allowed to use the swimming beach at Spruce Run Recreation Area.

Anglers can test their skills on the wild trout in Willoughby Brook. Chefs are not so lucky; all fish caught in the stream must be released. Children can fish in two ponds in the park, where bass and bluegill are often caught. Between September and January, two-thirds of the park is open to hunting that is subject to regulation. Check with a ranger.

If you visit Voorhees State Park on a summer weekend, be sure to visit the observatory. The Paul H. Robinson Observatory at the Edwin E. Aldrin Astronomical Center (named after Montclair native and second man on the moon "Buzz" Aldrin) opens its doors to the public on summer Saturday nights between 8:30 p.m. and 10:30 p.m. and on Sunday afternoons. Visitors may have the opportunity to look through a 26-inch telescope or through a number of smaller telescopes. Astronomers request that visitors dim their headlights upon entering the center's parking area. The public is also welcome to attend monthly meetings, which are held on the fourth Saturday of every month except December and January.

Voorhees State Park is a "carry in/carry out" park, as are many New Jersey public areas. Visitors are given trash bags when they enter the park and are asked to take their trash home for disposal. Campers can leave their rubbish and recycling in designated bins at the campground. Do not leave trash or food around your campsite or in your tent, and pay attention to warnings of bears. See the Introduction (page 2) for more information on how to camp safely in bear country.

Many of the trails, trees, and structures were built by the CCC in the 1930s, right after former Governor Voorhees donated his 325-acre farm to New Jersey. The Voorhees camp housed as many as 200 of Franklin Delano Roosevelt's "tree army," unemployed young men sent to remote areas to work on conserva-

KEY INFORMATION

ADDRESS:	Voorhees State Park 251 County Road 51 Glen Gardner, NJ 08826
OPERATED BY:	State Park Service
INFORMATION:	(908) 638-6969
WEB SITE:	www.njparksand forests.org
OPEN:	Year-round
SITES:	50
EACH SITE HAS:	Picnic table, fire ring
ASSIGNMENT:	First come, first served
REGISTRATION:	On arrival or reserve minimum 2 nights
FACILITIES:	Water, flush toilets, showers
PARKING:	At site, 2-vehicle limit
FEE:	$15
ELEVATION:	800 feet
RESTRICTIONS:	Pets: Prohibited Fires: In fire rings only Alcohol: Prohibited Vehicles: No limit; no hookups Other: Quiet hours 10 p.m.–6 a.m.; 14-night, 6-person, 2-tent limit

MAP

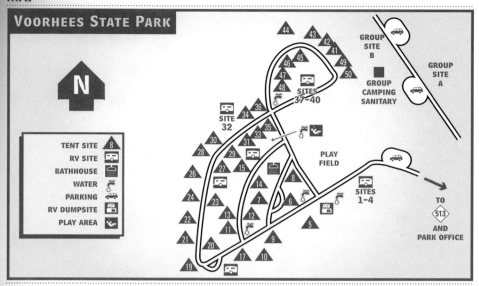

VOORHEES STATE PARK

N

TENT SITE	8
RV SITE	
BATHHOUSE	
WATER	
PARKING	
RV DUMPSITE	
PLAY AREA	

GROUP SITE B

GROUP SITE A

GROUP CAMPING SANITARY

SITES 37–40

SITE 32

PLAY FIELD

SITES 1–4

TO 513 AND PARK OFFICE

GETTING THERE

From I-78, exit at NJ 31 North. At the second traffic light, turn right onto CR 513 north through High Bridge. Follow the signs to the park.

tion projects as a response to the Great Depression. It was one of the most successful New Deal programs. Over the nine years it existed, the CCC built more than 40,000 bridges, planted 2 billion trees, improved or built thousands of structures and roads, and created 800 state parks.

FDR's army with shovels would be amazed today. While still suitably rustic and rural in appearance, Voorhees can no longer be considered remote. A New Jersey Transit train from the nearby picturesque town of High Bridge whisks daily commuters to Manhattan in an hour and a half.

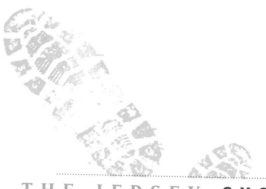

THE JERSEY **SHORE**

ATLANTIC CITY NORTH FAMILY CAMPGROUND

"**W**E CHASE ALL UNFAMILIAR** vehicles," reads the copy on the combination map/brochure you're handed at check-in at Atlantic City North Family Campground.

Security is nice to have, but it is hardly an issue at this private, wooded campground in the Pinelands. Fortunately, Atlantic City North offers more than just safety assurances. With all its amenities, including a store, rental cabins, RV sites, and Sunday morning pancake breakfast, the campground may seem like it offers too much to be included in a book on rustic tent sites.

Don't judge too quickly. Instead circle around from the main entrance past the camp store. Head straight to the western end of the grounds, where a triangular spur juts out from the main RV circle. The spur contains a pleasant surprise: a spacious, shady area dedicated solely to tenting.

Dogs, dog owners, and campers who prefer to be far away from dogs will appreciate the dedicated dog-walking path around the perimeter of the property. No hiking trails exist in the campground itself, but there are dozens of miles of hiking, biking, and equestrian trails in nearby Bass River State Forest. Dogs on leash are allowed in New Jersey state parks during the day but are prohibited from staying overnight, so dog owners must rely on private campgrounds if they want to bring the family pooch along for the ride.

The Batona Trail (Back To Nature Trail), a level 50-mile path through the Pinelands National Reserve, ends just north of Atlantic City North Family Campground. It was planned, cleared, and is maintained by the Batona Hiking Club in conjunction with the State Park Service. This easy wilderness trail passes animals, plants, ponds, and wild berries along the way under the Pine Barrens. The Batona Trail passes through Bass River State Forest, Wharton State Forest, and Brendan

> *High-season campers can sign up for a shuttle to and from Atlantic City.*

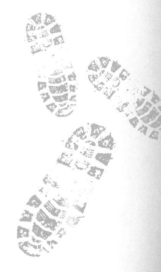

RATINGS

Beauty: ✿ ✿
Privacy: ✿ ✿
Spaciousness: ✿ ✿ ✿
Quiet: ✿ ✿
Security: ✿ ✿ ✿ ✿
Cleanliness: ✿ ✿ ✿

ADDRESS:	Atlantic City North Family Campground Stage Road Tuckerton, NJ 08087
OPERATED BY:	Private
INFORMATION:	(609) 296-9776
WEB SITE:	www.campacn.com
OPEN:	Year-round
SITES:	33 tent-only sites; 119 RV sites
EACH SITE HAS:	Picnic table, fire ring
ASSIGNMENT:	Choose from available sites
REGISTRATION:	On arrival at central office or reserve ahead
FACILITIES:	Water, flush toilets, showers, laundry, store, pay phone
PARKING:	At site; 2-vehicle limit
FEE:	$29
ELEVATION:	20 feet
RESTRICTIONS:	**Pets:** On leash **Fires:** In fire rings only; woodcutting prohibited **Alcohol:** Prohibited **Vehicles:** Up to 40 feet **Other:** Motorcycles must be walked into campground; quiet hours 11 p.m.–8 a.m.

T. Byrne State Forest. Remember, the Batona Trail is for hikers only. Mountain bikers, horses, and motorized vehicles are strictly prohibited.

Motorized vehicles are, however, welcome on the New Jersey Coastal Heritage Trail. It's an auto trail that invites visitors to journey along the southern and eastern coast of New Jersey, stopping en route at designated natural and historical sites. The trail stretches from Delaware Memorial Bridge at the southwestern tip of the state to Cape May on the southeastern peninsula to Perth Amboy, just south of Staten Island and the city of New York. Atlantic City North sits just outside the Barnegat Bay Region, known for not only its barrier islands but also for the beaches of Long Beach Island.

Although Atlantic City North is close to Atlantic City, it is not the closest tent campground: that honor belongs to Birch Grove Park. It does feature one amenity that trumps nearby competitors. High-season campers can sign up for a shuttle to and from Atlantic City. Check ahead for details; shuttles do not always run, and campers must stay a minimum of two nights to use this service.

Atlantic City is not just for gamblers. Its boardwalk, buffets, arcades, beach, and even its dollar stores can make for an enjoyable day out. It's all the more appealing for campers—when you tire of the glitz and casinos, you can return to your homey canvas estate under the Pineland stars.

Closer to the campground you will find the Edwin B. Forsythe National Wildlife Refuge, a 46,000-acre area comprised of wetlands, woodlands, and salt meadows. The refuge is divided into two distinct regions that are not connected, the Barnegat and the Brigantine regions. There is little public access into the refuge save for an 8-mile auto-tour route and two short nature trails. Two undeveloped barrier beaches here are dedicated to waterfowl and shorebirds—no access for humans.

For a deposit of $20, campers can borrow a beach badge from the campground. It must be returned to the campground staff at the end of the day. This allows campers onto Ship Bottom Beach at Long Beach Island. Children under age 12 and adults over age 65 are not required to have a badge.

MAP

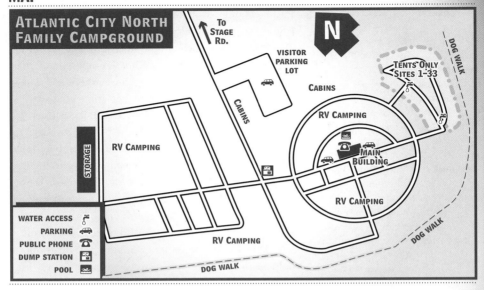

ATLANTIC CITY NORTH FAMILY CAMPGROUND

To STAGE RD.

VISITOR PARKING LOT

CABINS

CABINS

DOG WALK

TENTS ONLY SITES 1-33

RV CAMPING

RV CAMPING

MAIN BUILDING

STORAGE

RV CAMPING

RV CAMPING

DOG WALK

WATER ACCESS
PARKING
PUBLIC PHONE
DUMP STATION
POOL

DOG WALK

Also worth a visit is Tuckerton Seaport, a living-history museum dedicated to the heritage of the New Jersey shore region. Tuckerton Seaport features a working seaport village, sea captain's home, a 1930s houseboat, and most unexpectedly, two decoy shops.

More decoys are on display at the Noyes Museum of Art in Oceanville, south of Tuckerton on US 9. The Noyes Museum displays American fine and folk art with an emphasis on the southern Jersey region, but it is best known for its large collection of vintage duck decoys.

Atlantic City North Family Campground is ideally situated for more than duck decoys. It provides easy access to the Pinelands, the beach, and best of all, it has a nice tenting area where the family dog can join the fun.

GETTING THERE

From the Garden State Parkway, take Exit 58. Turn left onto County Road 539. Turn right onto Poor Man's Parkway. Drive 5 miles to Stage Road. Turn left, and the campground entrance is on the right after 1 mile.

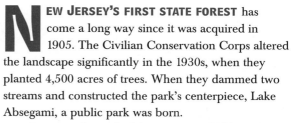

BASS RIVER STATE FOREST

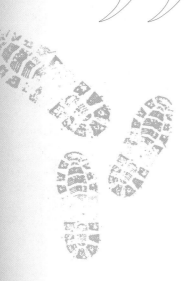

> *This century-old state forest in New Jersey features wooded camp-sites near a 67-acre lake.*

NEW JERSEY'S FIRST STATE FOREST has come a long way since it was acquired in 1905. The Civilian Conservation Corps altered the landscape significantly in the 1930s, when they planted 4,500 acres of trees. When they dammed two streams and constructed the park's centerpiece, Lake Absegami, a public park was born.

A century later, the lake is surrounded by 176 campsites, six cabins, six huts, nine primitive shelters, and six group sites. Eighty-three campsites line the thin loop that comprises the South Shore Campground. A separate loop sits on the farther bank, housing 93 additional sites at the North Shore Campground.

All sites are wooded, shady, and feature convenient access to modern facilities. Both loops have a central bathhouse that includes laundry and shower facilities in addition to sinks and toilets. None of the sites are lakefront, but cabins and huts sit on Lake Absegami's north shore. Campsites are level and spacious enough so that neighbors may be visible, but campers are not setting up tents on top of each other. Insects are savage here, so bring insecticide or be prepared to involuntarily feed them dinner. Note that the South Shore Campground sits within earshot of Stage Road, which vehicles use at all hours.

Bass River State forest is only a 20-minute drive from the seaside resort towns of Long Beach Island. Atlantic City is 25 miles to the southeast, but Bass River, with its swimming, boating, fishing, and trails, is a destination unto itself.

When lifeguards are on duty, swimming is allowed at the designated swimming beach on the eastern side of 67-acre Lake Absegami. Lifeguards usually patrol the swimming beach from 10 a.m. to 6 p.m. between Memorial Day weekend and Labor Day. Early in the season, the park staff recommends calling

RATINGS

Beauty: ✪ ✪ ✪ ✪
Privacy: ✪ ✪ ✪
Spaciousness: ✪ ✪ ✪ ✪ ✪
Quiet: ✪ ✪ ✪
Security: ✪ ✪ ✪
Cleanliness: ✪ ✪ ✪

ahead to confirm opening hours. The swimming beach complex includes a modern full-service bathhouse, first-aid station, refreshment stand, and beach supply concession. There is a playground nearby as well as picnic facilities and a parking lot. Both campgrounds are at least a half mile from the swimming beach. Campers do not have to pay admission to enter the swimming beach.

A summer rowboat concession and boat launch are also located near the swimming beach. Canoes and kayaks are available in nearby towns. Gas-powered engines are not allowed on Lake Absegami; power-boats are limited to using electric motors. Life pre-servers must be worn by occupants of all boats.

Five self-guided hiking trails are located near the campgrounds. They all begin in the parking lot near the swimming beach and vary in length from 1 mile to 3.2 miles. Additionally, a 0.5-mile trail runs from the entrance road through the 28-acre Absegami Natural Area. Here you can view a typical cross section of local pinelands. Oak and pine trees tower over a small white cedar bog. An interpretive center, located in the South Shore Campground, also provides information on the local ecosystem.

Other hiking trails are designated by colored blazes. The pink trail is the longest at 3.2 miles. It crosses Stage Road and passes the CCC/Forest Fire Service Memorial. The Bass River area has had at least four major fires. In 1936, five CCC workers died fighting a 58,000-acre fire near Bass River. In 1977, four volunteer firefighters died fighting a 2,300-acre fire in Bass River State Forest.

The 50-mile-long Batona Trail terminates near the South Shore Campground, at the intersection of Stage and Coal Roads. This level, easy wilderness trail tra-verses the Pinelands between Brendan T. Byrne State Park and Bass River State Forest. Horses and mountain bikes are prohibited on Batona Trail; it is for hikers only.

Miles of sand and gravel roads wind through the forest and are open to hiking, biking, horseback riding, and motorized vehicle use. Snowmobiles may use some of the roads in winter. Many roads are marked and can be found on the park map, available at the

KEY INFORMATION

ADDRESS:	Bass River State Forest 762 Stage Road New Gretna, NJ 08224
OPERATED BY:	State Park Service
INFORMATION:	(609) 296-1114
WEB SITE:	www.njparksand forests.org
OPEN:	Year-round
SITES:	176
EACH SITE HAS:	Picnic table, fire ring
ASSIGNMENT:	Choose from available sites
REGISTRATION:	On arrival or reserve minimum 2 nights
FACILITIES:	Water, flush toilets, showers, laundry
PARKING:	At site, 2-vehicle limit
FEE:	$15
ELEVATION:	20 feet
RESTRICTIONS:	Pets: Prohibited Fires: In fire rings only Alcohol: Prohibited Vehicles: No limit Other: Quiet hours 10 p.m.–6 a.m.; 14-night, 6-person, 2-tent limit

MAP

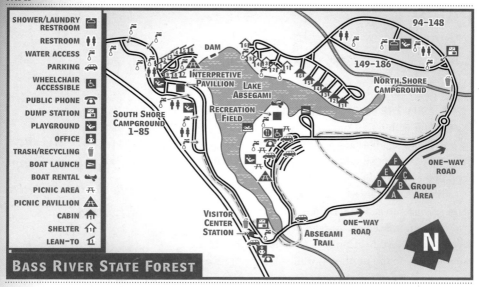

SHOWER/LAUNDRY RESTROOM
RESTROOM
WATER ACCESS
PARKING
WHEELCHAIR ACCESSIBLE
PUBLIC PHONE
DUMP STATION
PLAYGROUND
OFFICE
TRASH/RECYCLING
BOAT LAUNCH
BOAT RENTAL
PICNIC AREA
PICNIC PAVILLION
CABIN
SHELTER
LEAN-TO

149-186

NORTH SHORE CAMPGROUND

DAM

INTERPRETIVE PAVILLION

LAKE ABSEGAMI

SOUTH SHORE CAMPGROUND 1-85

RECREATION FIELD

F
E C
D B GROUP
A AREA

ONE-WAY ROAD

VISITOR CENTER STATION

ABSEGAMI TRAIL

ONE-WAY ROAD

N

BASS RIVER STATE FOREST

GETTING THERE

From the Garden State Parkway, take Exit 52. Take the ramp toward Batsto River–Bass River State Park. Go straight onto County Road 654. After 1 mile, turn right onto Stage Road. Follow Stage Road to the entrance on the left.

forest office. Some roads can be wet and muddy. Seek local information first; use caution and common sense before driving into the wilderness.

Fishing is allowed in Lake Absegami as well as in nearby streams and rivers. Pickerel, sunfish, and catfish have been caught at Bass River, but fish are not plentiful. Those age 16 or older must get a license before fishing. Both licenses and bait are available nearby.

During summer months, local nature groups and park personnel offer films and interpretive programs. In the past, offerings have included films, slideshows, stargazing evenings, and full-moon hikes. Information is provided on the Pinelands, Bass River, and the 3,830-acre West Pine Plains Natural Area, or Pygmy Pines, also found within the forest. Check with the park office for current information.

It's been over a hundred years since the state of New Jersey devoted its first efforts to Bass River State Forest. Today, the park is a model of success in the areas of public recreation, water conservation, wildlife, and forest management.

BIRCH GROVE PARK

EASILY THE MOST AFFORDABLE accommodation within the Atlantic City area, Birch Grove Park's shady sites offer a natural antidote for those sickened by gambling losses or by one too many zeppoli on the nearby boardwalk.

Birch Grove's forest is deceptive; its 271 wooded acres seem remote. The flashing lights and beach crowds seem miles away instead of just over Lakes Bay and the Northfield Bridge. Atlantic City is a 15-minute drive to the northeast, while Ocean City is a 15-minute drive in the opposite direction.

But no cities come to mind on the forested loops of Birch Grove Park's campground. The 50 sites have limited privacy from each other, but groves of woods protect them from the outside world. Both a pond and a lake sit on the outskirts. Plenty of RVs fit into the campground, and Birch Grove is a rare public park that does offer hookups. Pets are also allowed at the campground, although they cannot go into the main recreation area of the park; dogs tend to get excited at the vast number of ducks quacking about the central lake.

Golden Pond, across from the snack bar and office, is the park's centerpiece. It is surrounded by park benches, a trail, and hundreds of ducks. The central activity areas are all located nearby. A miniature golf course, playground, nature center, and picnic area are all across the road. Ball fields, a bandstand, and the Northfield Garden Club headquarters sit near the park entrance. The campground is within walking distance.

Nearly two dozen small ponds and lakes are situated throughout the park. Nature did not entirely plan this maze of scenic wetlands. From 1847 to 1951, the park was Somers Brick Yard. Clay and sand were mined from the soggy ground. Water rose to the surface, creating lakes where none had existed. In 1977, underground

> *Check into the most affordable accommodation in the Atlantic City area.*

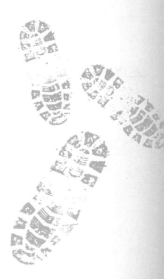

RATINGS

Beauty: ☆ ☆ ☆
Privacy: ☆ ☆ ☆
Spaciousness: ☆ ☆ ☆
Quiet: ☆ ☆ ☆
Security: ☆ ☆ ☆
Cleanliness: ☆ ☆ ☆

ADDRESS:	Birch Grove Park
	Burton Avenue
	Northfield, NJ 08225
OPERATED BY:	City of Northfield
INFORMATION:	(609) 641-3778
WEB SITE:	www.birchgrove
	park.org
OPEN:	April 1–
	mid-October
SITES:	51
EACH SITE HAS:	Picnic table, fire ring
ASSIGNMENT:	On arrival or by
	reservation
REGISTRATION:	On arrival or by
	reservation
FACILITIES:	Flush toilets, show-
	ers, water, laundry
PARKING:	At site; 2-vehicle
	maximum
FEE:	$18 per night, up to
	4 people
ELEVATION:	15 feet
RESTRICTIONS:	**Pets:** 2 per site;
	prohibited in rest of
	park
	Fires: In fire ring
	subject to
	restrictions
	Alcohol: Prohibited
	Vehicles: No limit
	Other: Must be over
	21 to register; maxi-
	mum 1-week stay

pipes were added to facilitate the movement of water and aquatic life between ponds. The environment is ideal for fish and wildlife and is now home to osprey, egrets, turtles, frogs, and herons. The municipal government has stated its dedication to preserving Birch Grove as a natural habitat and open space.

Birch Grove is a popular fishing spot, as several of 21 lakes are stocked with trout. Catfish, sunfish, largemouth bass, perch, and pike have also been caught here. Birch Grove is home to several annual fishing tournaments. Fishing requires a license for those over age 16; fishing for trout requires an additional fee and stamp.

Five miles of hiking trails wind through the woods and around the ponds. One trail is developed complete with Parcourse fitness stations. The other trails are more rugged. The last time a team counted, 599 species were identified as living in the park. Of these, many are threatened, such as the Pine Barrens tree frog and the short-eared owl.

The Birch Grove trail map comes with a warning: "The lake boundaries change according to the water level." Also, the sediment from the bottom is soft and sinks under the weight of people and animals. Stick to the trails. Exercise caution regarding ticks.

Events take place at Birch Grove throughout the summer. Bands play at the gazebo on designated Sundays and Tuesdays. The Nature Center hosts children's lectures on zoo animals, snakes, and ocean life. And the Northfield Garden Club hosts workshops on floral design and plants of the Pine Barrens.

If you tire of hiking, fishing, and mini-golf, hop in your car and take a ride to the shore. The casinos, beach, and boardwalk (the first in the world) are nearby in Atlantic City. If you're searching for activities that are a little more natural in scope, drive to Ocean City for a swim and then head south to Corson's Inlet State Park. Ocean City features 8 miles of guarded beaches. Corson's Inlet State Park's 350 acres are some of the last undeveloped acres along the Jersey Shore. Sunbathing, boating, hiking, and fishing are popular, but swimming is not allowed. Birders should note that the 98-acre Strathmere Natural Area within Corson's Inlet is a protected nesting area for shorebirds and waterfowl.

MAP

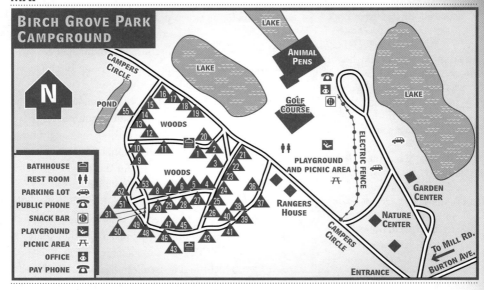

BIRCH GROVE PARK CAMPGROUND

LAKE

ANIMAL PENS

CAMPERS CIRCLE

LAKE

N

POND

16 15 17 18 19
55 14
13
12 WOODS
20

GOLF COURSE

LAKE

ELECTRIC FENCE

10 11 1 2 21
9 3 22
WOODS 23

PLAYGROUND AND PICNIC AREA

GARDEN CENTER

52 53 8 7 6 5 4 24 36
51 30 29 28 27 25 38 37
31 26 40 39
50 49 47 45
48 46 41
43 43

RANGERS HOUSE

NATURE CENTER

CAMPERS CIRCLE

To MILL RD.

BURTON AVE.

ENTRANCE

BATHHOUSE	
REST ROOM	
PARKING LOT	
PUBLIC PHONE	
SNACK BAR	
PLAYGROUND	
PICNIC AREA	
OFFICE	
PAY PHONE	

The Coastal Heritage Trail runs through Corson's Inlet, as does a suggested bicycle route that goes from Cape May to Ocean City. The Coastal Heritage Trail is an auto route that follows the coast from the Delaware Memorial Bridge to Cape May, and then travels north as far as Perth Amboy.

Those looking to stay a little closer to Birch Grove Park can visit Lucy the Elephant in Margate, directly across the Northfield Bridge from Northfield. Lucy is made of wood and tin, so it would be a stretch to consider her wildlife, but she has long been a roadside attraction. Standing 64 feet tall and weighing 90 tons, Lucy is a National Historic Landmark.

Birch Grove has no elephants and its petting zoo has closed, but it does feature ducks, fish, and some lovely shaded campsites. Take time out from the slot machines to relax in nature and enjoy the cheapest "rooms" in town.

GETTING THERE

From the Atlantic City Expressway, take Exit 7S to the Garden State Parkway South to Exit 36. Bear right onto Tilton Road and then make the first right onto Fire Road. Go left onto Mill Road at the third light. Follow Mill Road to Burton Avenue. Bear left. The park is on the left.

CEDAR CREEK CAMPGROUND

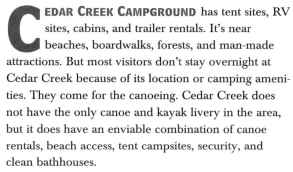

> *Most visitors come for the canoeing, but there are 45 shaded tent sites at Cedar Creek.*

CEDAR CREEK CAMPGROUND has tent sites, RV sites, cabins, and trailer rentals. It's near beaches, boardwalks, forests, and man-made attractions. But most visitors don't stay overnight at Cedar Creek because of its location or camping amenities. They come for the canoeing. Cedar Creek does not have the only canoe and kayak livery in the area, but it does have an enviable combination of canoe rentals, beach access, tent campsites, security, and clean bathhouses.

The 45 tent sites sit along the southern and western ends of the park, under hardwood trees. They are shaded and separate from the RV sites. Tent sites 1, 3, 7, 9, 11, 13, 14, and 15 are the closest of all 265 sites to Cedar Creek. All of the tent sites are near the canoe takeout point at Cedar Creek. Some are surrounded by understory nearby, while most are open to other sites.

Canoe and kayak trips are offered in three lengths; 6-, 12-, or 17-mile trips. Reservations during busy summer weekends are a must and are recommended at other times as well. The canoe livery is not open during winter. Boxed lunches are available and should be booked in advance. Note that while you can drink alcohol at your campsite, you cannot drink it in the canoes because the trips pass through New Jersey state parklands where alcohol consumption is prohibited. You do not have to rent a Cedar Creek canoe; if you bring your own, the staff will transport it for a fee.

The 6-mile trip provides a nice meandering hour-long journey along Cedar Creek, but the longer trips begin in Double Trouble State Park and take a minimum of three hours to complete. Cedar Creek's staff encourages paddlers to take their time and enjoy the trip, but all boats must be returned to the canoe livery by 6 p.m.

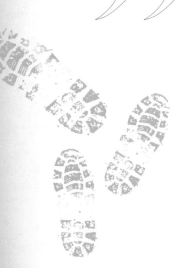

RATINGS

Beauty: ✿ ✿
Privacy: ✿ ✿
Spaciousness: ✿ ✿ ✿
Quiet: ✿ ✿ ✿
Security: ✿ ✿ ✿ ✿
Cleanliness: ✿ ✿ ✿

Double Trouble State Park is a 7,000-acre typical Pinelands forest, complete with a historic village and cranberry bogs. Cedar Creek is sometimes narrow, but its waters flow quickly and can be an excellent run for inexperienced canoeists. Keep your eyes open, and in addition to cranberry bogs and Pinelands plants, you might see deer, beavers, otters, or birds. The park also features multiuse trails, fishing, and cedar swamps. It is a designated stop on the 300-mile auto route called the New Jersey Coastal Heritage Trail Route.

If you prefer saltwater and sailing to canoeing under pine trees, cross US 9 and drive a half mile east to Cedar Creek Marina. Barnegat Bay Sail Charters offers both sailing lessons and sailboat rentals. Afternoon or sunset sail cruises are available, letting the crew do the work while you enjoy the ocean views.

For those with energy left after a day of canoeing, the boardwalk thrills of Seaside Heights are only 15 miles away. Leave the peaceful forest behind and head to the mile-long boardwalk for some electronically powered fun at the arcades, carnival rides, miniature golf, fast-food stands, and antique carousel of this shore resort.

Just south of Seaside Heights, but more suited to a daylight visit, is Island Beach State Park. The 3,000 acres of 10-mile-long Island Beach State Park have been deliberately undeveloped and feature one of the longest remaining stretches of barrier beach along the northern Atlantic Coast. One mile of the park is open to swimmers during the summer, with bathhouses and parking—concessions to modern life among this natural environment. Scuba diving, saltwater fishing, and surfing are also allowed at Island Beach. Additionally, the park features a 5-mile bike path, hiking trails, horseback riding trails, and a bird observation blind.

Immediately south of Island Beach, at the northern tip of Long Beach Island, is Barnegat Lighthouse State Park. The lighthouse is no longer in service and has been a state park since the 1950s. Both the lighthouse and its interpretive center were renovated in 2003. Climb the 217 lighthouse steps for a panoramic view of the ocean and surrounding beaches or take a

ADDRESS:	Cedar Creek Campground 1052 US 9 Bayville, NJ 08721
OPERATED BY:	Private
INFORMATION:	(732) 269-1413
WEB SITE:	www.cedarcreeknj.com
OPEN:	Year-round
SITES:	45 tent; 220 RV
EACH SITE HAS:	Picnic table, fire ring
ASSIGNMENT:	Choose from available sites
REGISTRATION:	On arrival or by reservation
FACILITIES:	Water, flush toilets, showers, laundry, store, pay phone
PARKING:	At site; 1-car limit per site
FEE:	$28 for 2; each child age 16 and younger, $3; each additional adult, $17
ELEVATION:	40 feet
RESTRICTIONS:	Pets: On leash Fires: In fire ring Alcohol: At site Vehicles: No limit Other: No profane language or intoxication; quiet hours 11 p.m.–7 a.m.

MAP

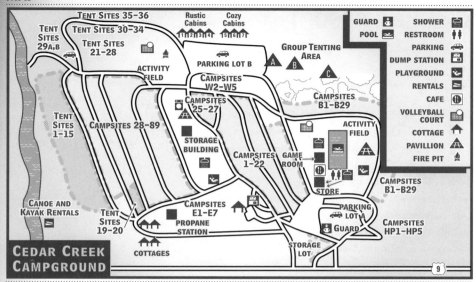

CEDAR CREEK CAMPGROUND

Tent Sites 35–36
Tent Sites 30–34
Tent Sites 21–28
Tent Sites 29A,B
Rustic Cabins
Cozy Cabins
ACTIVITY FIELD
PARKING LOT B
CAMPSITES W2–W5
Tent Sites 1–15
CAMPSITES 28–89
CAMPSITES 25–27
STORAGE BUILDING
CAMPSITES 1–22
GAME ROOM
GROUP TENTING AREA
A B C
CAMPSITES B1–B29
ACTIVITY FIELD
STORE
CAMPSITES B1–B29
CANOE AND KAYAK RENTALS
TENT SITES 19–20
CAMPSITES E1–E7
PROPANE STATION
COTTAGES
STORAGE LOT
PARKING LOT A
GUARD
CAMPSITES HP1–HP5

GUARD
POOL
SHOWER
RESTROOM
PARKING
DUMP STATION
PLAYGROUND
RENTALS
CAFE
VOLLEYBALL COURT
COTTAGE
PAVILLION
FIRE PIT

9

GETTING THERE

From the Garden State Parkway southbound, take Exit 80. Bear right onto US 9 South. Drive 6.5 miles south to the campground on the right.

short walk through the park on the Maritime Forest Trail, perfect for viewing the environment that once would have been found all along the coast.

Closer beaches to Cedar Creek Campground include Berkeley Island County Park and William J. Dudley Park. The latter is just south of the campground and features barbecue areas and a roller hockey rink along with a swimming area. Twenty-five-acre Berkeley Island County Park is 2 miles west of Cedar Creek on a Barneget Bay peninsula, and has a fishing and crabbing pier in addition to a beach. Both parks are in protected Barnegat Bay, not directly on the Atlantic Ocean.

Cedar Creek Campground may not be the ideal spot for someone searching for a deserted forest campsite. But for families or groups looking for a wide variety of activities, Cedar Creek has a versatile list of offerings from beach access to marshmallow roasts to peaceful paddling trips through Double Trouble State Park.

NORTH WILDWOOD CAMPING RESORT

THE **CAPE MAY PENINSULA** is 16 miles long, 8 miles wide, and features more than a dozen campgrounds. Many more line US 9 north of the peninsula. Nearly all of these campgrounds densely pack in RVs; almost none are tent friendly. Most encourage seasonal camping. Some don't even allow tent camping. North Wildwood Camping Resort is not included here because it has the most pristine, rustic, wilderness sites in the Garden State. It is included here because it has a tent section and is therefore a beacon of light amongst the glut of southern coastal RV parks.

The RV section of North Wildwood looks similar to neighboring campgrounds, but continue driving past the 11 small hookup lanes to the very end. A small, dedicated tenting loop sits on a northern spur apart from the other sites. There is no underbrush between sites, but there are trees and shade above the tents. Tent campers are not shoved in amongst the RVs here; they have their own real estate and are given the respect they miss at many RV parks.

Dogs are allowed to come camping, too, but cannot be left unattended at campsites. A small area solely for dog walking lies at the southwestern end of the campground. Dog owners are required to clean up after their pets. The campground features the usual amenities found in private parks, such as a pool, store, playground, and a few game courts. But campsites and comfort take precedence over organized activities.

North Wildwood Camping Resort is actually located in Cape May Court House, 5 miles from the Wildwoods. North Wildwood, Wildwood, and Wildwood Crest make up the Wildwoods and are located on New Jersey's southernmost barrier island. Beach access is free along the 5 miles of coast, a rarity on the Jersey Shore (Atlantic City's beach also has no admission charge).

> *North Wildwood features the only tent sites on the Cape May peninsula.*

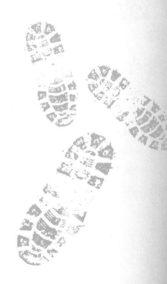

RATINGS

Beauty: ✿ ✿
Privacy: ✿ ✿
Spaciousness: ✿ ✿ ✿
Quiet: ✿ ✿
Security: ✿ ✿ ✿ ✿
Cleanliness: ✿ ✿ ✿

ADDRESS: North Wildwood Camping Resort 240 West Shellbay Avenue Cape May Court House, NJ 08210

OPERATED BY: Private

INFORMATION: (609) 465-4440

WEB SITE: www.nwcamp.com

OPEN: April 15–Oct. 15

SITES: 33 tent; 234 RV

EACH SITE HAS: Picnic table, fire ring

ASSIGNMENT: Choose from available sites; requests not guaranteed

REGISTRATION: On arrival or by reservation

FACILITIES: Water, flush toilets, showers, laundry, store, pay phone

PARKING: At site; 1-car limit per site

FEE: 2 people, $31; children ages 2–17, $2; children ages 18–22, $4; adult, $17.50; seniors, $6

ELEVATION: 20 feet

RESTRICTIONS: Pets: On leash Fires: In fire rings; no woodcutting Alcohol: At site Vehicles: No limit Other: Quiet hours 11 p.m.–8 a.m.

A preservation group and the Greater Wildwoods Tourism Authority have said that the Wildwoods claim to fame is its "large collection of mid-century doo-wop architecture." In layman's terms, this means the Wildwoods had a boom during the 1950s. Hotels and clubs were built, and entertainers visited the town. Some nicknamed Wildwood "Little Las Vegas." Chubby Checker debuted "The Twist" here, and the first national broadcast of *American Bandstand* was aired from Wildwood.

The moment passed, and Wildwood went down in history as a resort area past its prime. The beachfront property was ignored long enough so that when the area became desirable again, enough time had passed that the "doo-wop architecture" was preserved instead of destroyed, thanks to the efforts of the preservation group and local citizens. Pick up a map at the Doo-Wop Preservation League headquarters at Pine and Pacific avenues or join one of their trolley tours. You can see the boomerang roofs, faux Chinese temples, tiki-style shops, wacky neon signs, and kidney-shaped pools that were once state-of-the-art in Eisenhower's America. The largest concentration of these cool-turned-tacky-turned-kitsch retro buildings is in Wildwood Crest.

Wildwood has a 2-mile boardwalk that features piers full of amusement rides but is not known solely for its man-made attractions. Besides the free beach, which is getting bigger every year due to the southern movement of the sand, there are excellent opportunities for crabbing, whale-watching, and dolphin-watching.

A ten-minute ride south down the Garden State Parkway or US 9 takes campers from the 1950s to the 1850s. Cape May is best known not for its lovely beaches or migratory birds, but for its historic collection of Victorian-era buildings and its historic lighthouse. But there is more to Cape May than its architecture. Visit Cape May Point State Park and Cape May Migratory Bird Refuge. The peninsula is a major feeding and resting place for migratory birds. Cape May Point State Park contains a variety of habitats that nature lovers and birds both enjoy.

Bird-watchers don't even have to drive the 10 miles from North Wildwood Camping Resort to Cape

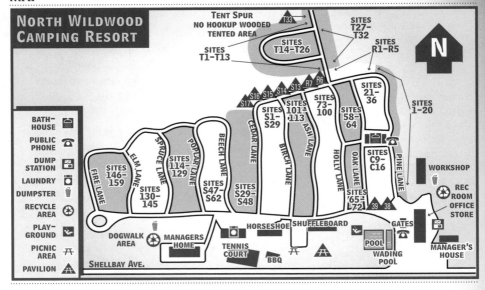

North Wildwood Camping Resort

TENT SPUR NO HOOKUP WOODED TENTED AREA

SITES T14–T26

SITES T1–T13

T33

SITES T27–T32

SITES R1–R5

N

R6

R7

S13 S14 S15 S16

S17

SITES 21–36

SITES 1–20

SITES S1–S29

SITES 101–113

SITES 73–100

SITES 58–64

BATH-HOUSE

PUBLIC PHONE

DUMP STATION

LAUNDRY

DUMPSTER

RECYCLE AREA

PLAY-GROUND

PICNIC AREA

PAVILION

SITES 146–159

SITES 114–129

SITES 130–145

SITES S47–S62

SITES S29–S48

SITES C9–C16

SITES 65–72

39 38

FIRE LANE

ELM LANE

SPRUCE LANE

POPLAR LANE

BEECH LANE

CEDAR LANE

BIRCH LANE

ASH LANE

HOLLY LANE

OAK LANE

PINE LANE

WORKSHOP

REC ROOM

OFFICE STORE

DOGWALK AREA

MANAGERS HOME

TENNIS COURT

BBQ

HORSESHOE

SHUFFLEBOARD

POOL

WADING POOL

GATES

MANAGER'S HOUSE

SHELLBAY AVE.

May to get a look at the tens of thousands of birds that stop over on the Cape May peninsula. Instead, they can drive a few miles north to Stone Harbor Bird Sanctuary, a municipal 21-acre heron sanctuary given landmark status by the National Park Service.

Stone Harbor is also home to the Wetlands Institute, a 34-acre salt marsh that celebrates the marsh, the surrounding beaches and wetlands, and wildlife. Exhibits include hands-on aquariums and live turtle exhibits. If you can tear the kids away from the Wildwood boardwalk, there are children and family interpretive programs at the Wetlands Institute during the summer.

North Wildwood Camping Resort may not feature bushy privacy barriers between sites or miles of hiking trails. But it does have the advantage of proximity to dozens of seashore attractions, both natural and man-made.

GETTING THERE

From the Garden State Parkway, take Exit 9 and go 1 mile west on Shellbay Avenue to the entrance on the right.

RIVERWOOD PARK

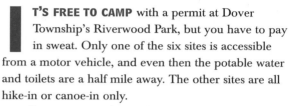

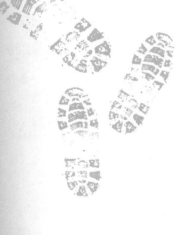

> *Canoeing and fishing are popular at these free, wooded riverside sites.*

IT'S FREE TO CAMP with a permit at Dover Township's Riverwood Park, but you have to pay in sweat. Only one of the six sites is accessible from a motor vehicle, and even then the potable water and toilets are a half mile away. The other sites are all hike-in or canoe-in only.

Campsites stretch out along 2 miles of eastern shoreline of the North Branch of the Toms River. Amenities vary by site. Some have brick fireplaces, trash cans, or benches, but all the Dover Township Department of Parks guarantees is the presence of a picnic table.

In spite of efforts to keep the park clean, litter tends to show up along the shoreline and near picnic tables. The park is still pleasant and wooded, with sites sitting far apart in private clearings among thick underbrush. The two sites at the northern end of the park are almost never used. The site at the end of Edgemere Road, termed "Kiwanis Campsite," is used frequently as it is only 120 steps from the second parking area. Edgemere Road is the next street north of the park's main entrance. Follow it to the end and then turn right onto a single-lane dirt road to reach the Kiwanis Campsite as well as the two seldom-used sites. Canoes can easily be pulled out of the river here, allowing canoeists an easy and legal night of camping as long as permits are obtained in advance.

Camping permits must be applied for at the main office of the Dover Township Parks Department. This is about 7 miles from Riverwood Park and must be scouted out in advance. The office is at 1810 Warren Point Road, off Fischer Boulevard by the bay in Toms River. From Exit 88 of the Garden State Parkway, head left on NJ 70 to Shorrock Street. Turn right onto Shorrock and then turn right onto County Road 549. Go right onto Fischer (CR 549 spur) and then go left

RATINGS

Beauty: ☆ ☆ ☆
Privacy: ☆ ☆ ☆ ☆
Spaciousness: ☆ ☆ ☆
Quiet: ☆ ☆ ☆
Security: ☆ ☆
Cleanliness: ☆ ☆

onto Merrimac. Warren Point Road is at the end of Merrimac. The office is open weekdays from 9 a.m. to 4 p.m.

Riverwood Park is a long, thin park that stretches along about 2 miles of riverfront and is no more than a half mile wide at its thickest point. Nevertheless, Dover Township has managed to fit in 2.5 miles of forest trails, three picnic areas, soccer fields, and a playground for children with disabilities. The playground was rebuilt in 2001 by inmates from Wrightstown's Mid-State Correctional Facility as part of the Community Labor Assistance Program. Even with all the amenities, the park still feels rural and wooded.

Fishing is popular in the Toms River along Riverwood Park. Trout are stocked several times a season. Some sites are right on the bank, and you could fish in your pajamas without even getting out of bed in the morning. Canoeing is also popular but somewhat challenging because the river is shallow and winds sharply at several points. Canoeing south from Riverwood takes canoeists near Surf and Stream Campground, past Albocondo Campground (which has a small tenting section), and finally through Winding River Park.

Dover Township also oversees Winding River Park, a 500-acre property of which only 40 acres are developed. Canoeists follow the river alongside the park for 6 miles. No camping is allowed at Winding River Park, but visitors can easily reach it from Riverwood, Surf and Stream, or Albocondo. Winding River features 8 miles of hiking trails, 3 miles of bike way, picnic areas, softball and soccer fields, equestrian trails, and an ice/roller skating rink.

To drive to Winding River Park from Riverwood Park, turn right onto Whitesville Road (CR 527). After 2 miles, turn left onto CR 571/Indian Head Road and then right onto Oak Ridge Parkway to Winding River Park.

Those interested in less natural pastimes can drive either 15 minutes to mega-amusement park Great Adventure or 10 miles in the other direction to Seaside Heights, an old-style Jersey Shore beach and boardwalk area that features carnival games and recreation.

KEY INFORMATION

ADDRESS:	Riverwood Park Riverwood Drive Toms River, NJ 08755
OPERATED BY:	Dover Township Department of Parks, Recreation, and Public Lands
INFORMATION:	(732) 341-1000, ext. 8415
WEB SITE:	www.townshipof dover.com/recreat. htm
OPEN:	Year-round
SITES:	6
EACH SITE HAS:	Picnic table
ASSIGNMENT:	At office
REGISTRATION:	Permit must be obtained in person
FACILITIES:	Flush toilets
PARKING:	At central lot; hike to sites
FEE:	Free
ELEVATION:	40 feet
RESTRICTIONS:	Pets: On leash Fires: Prohibited; us camp stoves Alcohol: Prohibited Vehicles: None Other: Permits can only be obtained weekdays 9 a.m.– 4 p.m.

MAP

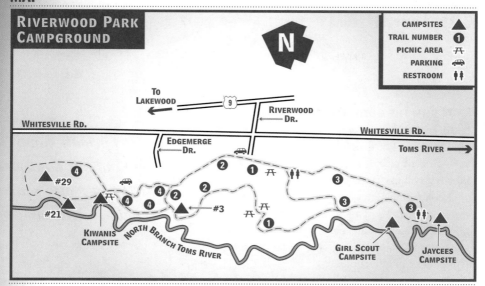

RIVERWOOD PARK CAMPGROUND

N

CAMPSITES ▲
TRAIL NUMBER ❶
PICNIC AREA ⊼
PARKING 🚐
RESTROOM 👫

To LAKEWOOD ←
9
RIVERWOOD DR.
WHITESVILLE RD.
WHITESVILLE RD.
EDGEMERGE DR. ←
TOMS RIVER →

▲ #29
▲ ⊼
#21
KIWANIS CAMPSITE
NORTH BRANCH TOMS RIVER

❷ ❶ ⊼ 👫
❷
❷ ❹ ❷
❹ ❹
❹ ❹ ▲ #3 ⊼ ⊼
❶

❸
❸
❸ 👫 ▲
▲
GIRL SCOUT CAMPSITE
JAYCEES CAMPSITE

GETTING THERE

From the Garden State Parkway, take Exit 88. Follow NJ 70 west for approximately 4 miles to Whitesville Road/CR 527. Turn left and continue for about 3 miles to Riverwood Drive. Turn right to the park.

South of Seaside Heights is Island Beach State Park, a sandy 3,000-acre undeveloped barrier beach known for its saltwater fishing and ocean swimming.

Riverwood is also a good base for a side trip to Double Trouble State Park, 10 miles south. Double Trouble is a 7,300-acre Pinelands forest that features 12 miles of hiking trails and 10 miles of Cedar Creek, which is popular with canoeists and kayakers. Double Trouble is best known for its historic village. Fourteen buildings from the late 1800s still stand in the village, including a general store, schoolhouse, cottages, and sawmill. Double Trouble was a cranberry farm and sawmill. Cranberries are still harvested in Double Trouble State Park, on lands leased from New Jersey.

Few people know that camping is allowed in Riverwood Park. For those willing to rough it, the campsites are ideal for the outdoors enthusiast on a budget.

SURF AND STREAM CAMPGROUND

FROM THE OUTSIDE, Surf and Stream Campground looks like another in a long line of generic RV parks that are located near the shore. Dozens of trailers are packed into a large loop that circles a busy recreation area.

Look a little closer, and you'll start to notice a bit more character. Many of Surf and Stream's clients are longtime repeat seasonal customers—not what you'd expect from a campground located close to some of the region's top attractions.

But the most unexpected perk of Surf and Stream is not its quirky cast of characters or its amenities or its live weekend music. It's a small, wooded island that is devoted solely to walk-in tent camping.

Tenters must park their cars nearby and carry their gear across a narrow wooden footbridge. Campground rules allow dogs (on leashes), but they are not allowed on the tenting island so be sure to leave them at home. There are no specific "sites," but there are a number of clearings on the island. Campers can pick an open area to be near other campers or can make their way to a private area on the island's tip. Plenty of picnic tables and grills are available, so drag them over to your space in the woods and designate it a site for the night.

Modern restrooms are a short walk away, back over the bridge. Water spigots are located on either end of the island. The central recreation area also features a miniature golf course, basketball court, swimming pool, volleyball court, and horseshoe pit. The main building includes a store, recreation hall, snack bar, laundry room, and adult lounge. It is possible to fish from the dock or riverbank. Catfish, pickerel, and bass have been caught in the river, a branch of the Toms. Canoeists can rent canoes (transportation included) at nearby Albocondo Campground.

> *This private campground has a wooded island devoted solely walk-in tent camping*

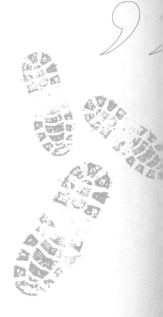

RATINGS

Beauty: ✿ ✿ ✿
Privacy: ✿ ✿ ✿
Spaciousness: ✿ ✿ ✿ ✿
Quiet: ✿ ✿ ✿
Security: ✿ ✿ ✿ ✿
Cleanliness: ✿ ✿ ✿

ADDRESS: Surf and Stream
Campground
1801 Ridgeway Road
Toms River, NJ
08757

OPERATED BY: Private

INFORMATION: (732) 349-8919

WEB SITE: www.surfnstream.
com

OPEN: Year-round

SITES: Open area, 30-tent
limit

EACH SITE HAS: Picnic table, grill

ASSIGNMENT: First come, first
served

REGISTRATION: At office; no reservations for tent island

FACILITIES: Water, flush toilets,
showers, laundry,
store, pay phone

PARKING: At central parking
area

FEE: Minimum, $27; adult,
$16; child, $4

ELEVATION: 25 feet

RESTRICTIONS: Pets: Prohibited on
island
Fires: In fire rings
Alcohol: At site only
Vehicles: None on
tent island
Other: Must be 21 or
older to register

Albocondo, located nearby at 1480 Whitesville Road, has 43 tenting spots among its 189 campsites. Most of the clean, spacious sites are located in the southern corner of the grounds, in a relatively private area. Showers are nearby. Pets are permitted to camp with owners at Albocondo.

Families traveling with children (and adults who like roller coasters) should note that mega-theme park Six Flags Great Adventure is 15 miles from Surf and Stream Campground. Next door to the theme park is a 45-acre water park and the world's largest drive-thru animal preserve outside of national parks in Africa. For those who prefer deer to rhino, the campground is also located near Pinelands National Reserve.

Many campers who visit Surf and Stream are there for the easy access to the sea. The Atlantic Ocean and Seaside Heights are only 10 miles away.

Seaside Heights, together with its less famous neighbor Seaside Park, is a major beach and recreation destination. The Seaside Heights boardwalk and pier is crowded with thrill rides, arcades, snack bars, and carnival games. Casino Pier, at the northern end, is renowned for its lovingly restored turn-of-the-century carousel. Some of the attractions have seen better days—the boardwalk is, after all, over 60 years old, but the frenetic pace of the boardwalk at night continues to attract fun seekers from all over New Jersey. Both towns offer beach access, but you must pay fees on weekends and designated days of the week. Parking is difficult, and visitors must use high-priced lots.

Seaside Heights is located on the Barnegat barrier island, one of several that protects the mainland Jersey coast. To avoid the crowds and hubbub of the boardwalk, head south down to Island Beach State Park.

The 9.5 miles of dunes and white sandy beaches of Island Beach State Park stand in stark contrast to the commercialism and frenzied pace of Seaside Heights. Its 3,000 mostly undeveloped acres give visitors an idea of how the shore used to be when it was in its natural state. One mile of the beach, in the center of the park, is designated for swimming. Lifeguards patrol the area during the summer. Parking, a bathhouse, and a snack bar are nearby.

MAP

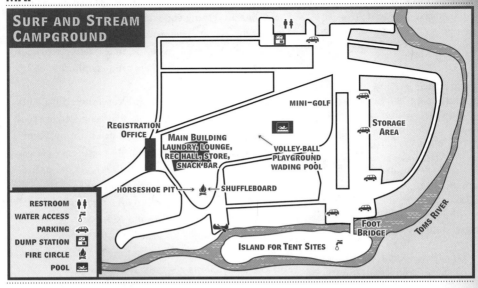

There is a natural area on either end of the beach. Access to the 659-acre Northern Natural Area is restricted. Both the Northern and 1,237-acre Southern Natural Area house a wide variety of wildlife, including New Jersey's largest osprey colony. There are bird observation blinds, and in summer visitors may observe wildlife from naturalist-guided canoe and kayak tours. Eight trails wind through the park. Scuba diving, fishing, sailing, and surfing are allowed at Island Beach. Check with the visitor center for regulations and locations.

Surf and Stream does not offer hiking paths and horseback trails like the state parks, but its tenting island is a gem among private parks, especially those nearest the shore.

GETTING THERE

From the north on the Garden State Parkway, take Exit 88 to NJ 70 West. Go right on NJ 70 for 6 miles. Turn left onto County Road 527 for 2.7 miles. Turn right onto CR 571. The entrance is on the left.

New Gretna

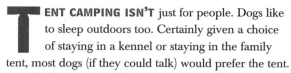

TIMBERLINE LAKE CAMPING RESORT

> *Campers can bring their dogs without giving up the seclusion and rustic atmosphere of a tent environment.*

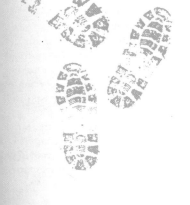

TENT CAMPING ISN'T just for people. Dogs like to sleep outdoors too. Certainly given a choice of staying in a kennel or staying in the family tent, most dogs (if they could talk) would prefer the tent.

No New Jersey state park allows dogs to stay overnight. Only a few municipal and county parks do not completely prohibit pets. Private campgrounds are often the only option for campers traveling with the furriest member of the family. Timberline Lake, ideally located in the Pinelands near the shore, offers the best compromise for families looking to camp with their dogs without giving up the seclusion and rustic atmosphere of a tenting environment. The tenting area is wooded, secure, and isolated from the denser RV area.

The 14 tent sites are located in the woods surrounding three sides of a large recreation field. Most sites are open to the other tent sites and to the field, but the woods provide a buffer between campers and the activity section of the campground. A trail connects the tenting area to the activity area, and a short gravel road leads to the office and bathhouse. The tent area itself is considered primitive, with portable toilets and no water faucets. Water must be carried in from the office area.

Reservations are only necessary on holiday weekends. Lakefront sites are also available to tent campers. They feature electric and water hookups, so expect to have RVs as neighbors if you opt for a site with a water view.

The lakeside beach is guarded and open to swimmers during the day on weekends. The swimming pool is open daily during summer months. Campers can rent canoes on weekends, and recreational equipment is available at the office. In exchange for a deposit, campers can borrow bats, baseballs, gloves, volleyballs, basketballs, footballs, horseshoes, and soccer balls. Be warned that the ball field is also the tent campers front

RATINGS

Beauty: ✿ ✿
Privacy: ✿ ✿ ✿
Spaciousness: ✿ ✿ ✿
Quiet: ✿ ✿ ✿
Security: ✿ ✿ ✿ ✿
Cleanliness: ✿ ✿ ✿

yard, so expect to have some company during the afternoons. Ping-pong is free in the store game room, provided you buy a twenty-five-cent ball. Fishing is popular in the 30-acre lake.

Kids will appreciate the campground's organized activities. In addition to sporting events, there is a weekly hayride, the occasional ice cream social, "Christmas in July," and beach games. Adult activities include bingo and horseshoe tournaments. The remote tenting area makes it easy for tent campers to avoid the organized fun and enjoy a more primitive experience.

Visitors can enjoy other activities at nearby Bass River State Forest, where park personnel offer interpretive programs and films. Past programs have included stargazing and full moon hikes through local Pinelands trails.

Timberline Lake Camping Resort sits squarely in the middle of the Pinelands, the unique ecological region that covers 1.1 million acres of southern Jersey. Bass River's hiking trails that wind through the forest's 27,000 acres are open to campers. Vehicle entrance fees are charged.

The 50-mile-long Batona Trail ends near the campground, in Bass River State Forest near the intersection of Stage and Coal roads. Hiking this level, easy trail is a great way to get to know the plants and animals of the Pinelands.

For beach lovers, Long Beach Island is a half-hour drive away. It's one of the best-known barrier islands along the Jersey Shore. Beach badges, or passes, must be purchased during the summer; costs vary from $3 to $7 per day. The northern tip of the island features Barnegat Lighthouse State Park. The 172-foot-tall Barnegat Lighthouse is open throughout the year and features panoramic views of the region. You can reach all of the Long Beach Island towns from NJ 72, a causeway that intersects with both US 9 and the Garden State Parkway.

A half-hour drive in the other direction will take you south to the casinos and beaches of Atlantic City. Even if you're not a gambler, it's worth visiting for the lights and atmosphere of the busy boardwalk (the world's first).

ADDRESS: Timberline Lake Camping Resort 365 County Road 67 New Gretna, NJ 08224

OPERATED BY: Private

INFORMATION: (609) 296-7900

WEB SITE: www.timberlinelake.com

OPEN: May 1–mid October

SITES: 14 tent sites

EACH SITE HAS: Picnic table, fire ring

ASSIGNMENT: On arrival or reserve 2 nights minimum

REGISTRATION: At office

FACILITIES: Portable toilets; office and RV area has water, flush toilets, showers, laundry, store, pay phone

PARKING: At site, 2-vehicle limit

FEE: $30

ELEVATION: 20 feet

RESTRICTIONS: Pets: On leash
Fires: In fire rings; no woodcutting
Alcohol: Permitted
Vehicles: Up to 35 feet
Other: After office hours, campers must use gate card; $10 deposit for card

MAP

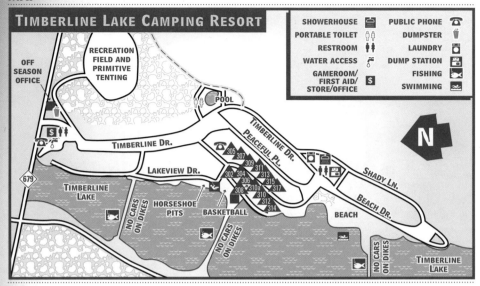

TIMBERLINE LAKE CAMPING RESORT

SHOWERHOUSE		PUBLIC PHONE	
PORTABLE TOILET		DUMPSTER	
RESTROOM		LAUNDRY	
WATER ACCESS		DUMP STATION	
GAMEROOM/ FIRST AID/ STORE/OFFICE	S	FISHING	
		SWIMMING	

OFF SEASON OFFICE

RECREATION FIELD AND PRIMITIVE TENTING

POOL

TIMBERLINE DR.

PEACEFUL PL.

TIMBERLINE DR.

SHADY LN.

LAKEVIEW DR.

305 307
309
311
302 304 306 313
308 310a 315
310 317
312
314

BEACH DR.

TIMBERLINE LAKE

NO CARS ON DIKES

HORSESHOE PITS

BASKETBALL

NO CARS ON DIKES

BEACH

NO CARS ON DIKES

TIMBERLINE LAKE

679

N

GETTING THERE

From the Garden State Parkway southbound, take Exit 52. Turn left onto US 9 then right at the light to CR 679. Drive 4 miles to Timberline Lake.

If the crowds of the casinos, shore, and the bingo games back at camp are too much for you, take some time out at the Edwin B. Forsythe National Wildlife Refuge. Its 40,000 acres include tidal salt meadows and marshes, preserved for use by migratory shorebirds, woodland trees and plants, and upland species. The refuge is split into two divisions: the Barnegat and Brigantine divisions. There are few hiking paths because it is a refuge dedicated to wildlife and not to humans. View the refuge from your car as you drive the 8-mile auto trail—stop to read the brochure at viewpoints.

Timberline Lake Camping Resort is ideally situated for access to the wildlife refuge, Pinelands, and shore. But its best feature is that it allows primitive tent camping for both people and dogs, but developed facilities are never far away.

SOUTHERN NEW JERSEY

ATLANTIC COUNTY PARK AT ESTELL MANOR

Mays Landing

IF YOU'RE LOOKING FOR CONVENIENCE, comfort, and small luxuries such as hot showers and well-marked roads, don't come to the camping area at Estell Manor. However, if you're hoping to get away from it all while not disappearing too far into the bush, this is the place for you. The campground at Atlantic County Park at Estell Manor is utterly off the beaten path but is still accessible to those on an overnight trip. It is not the sort of campground you would stumble over. In fact, it's hard to find even when following a map.

Campers must reserve sites in person at the Lake Lenape boathouse or by phone and mail. Call to have an application sent to you. The reservation office closes at 5 p.m. during spring and autumn; closing time is at 9 p.m. throughout summer. Don't leave Lake Lenape and drive to the developed loop road at Estell Manor. No, ask for a map and directions because the Estell Manor campground is located off tiny Artesian Well Road, the next turnoff north from the main park road.

The camping area is secure by default; only those aware of its existence would think to look for it here. But it is not within a guarded region or fence. Visitors must loop left off Artesian Well Road (there is a sign) and look for a gate. The camping area is located on a spur off the loop, behind the gate. Sites are level, spacious, sandy, and totally secluded. The area is popular with boaters because a ramp into the South River is located right next door. (Boaters must adhere to state boating regulations.) Facilities are limited to a portable toilet. A second portable toilet sits on Artesian Well Road, across from the group camping site.

The 2-mile Swamp Trail Boardwalk begins across Artesian Well Road from the loop that leads to the campsites. The boardwalk is for use exclusively by hik-

> *If you're hoping to get away from it all while not disappearing into the bush, stay at Estell Manor.*

RATINGS

Beauty: ✪ ✪ ✪ ✪
Privacy: ✪ ✪ ✪ ✪
Spaciousness: ✪ ✪ ✪ ✪ ✪
Quiet: ✪ ✪ ✪ ✪ ✪
Security: ✪ ✪
Cleanliness: ✪ ✪

120 THE BEST IN TENT CAMPING NEW JERSEY

ADDRESS:	Atlantic County Park at Estell Manor 109 NJ 50 Mays Landing, NJ 08330
OPERATED BY:	Atlantic County Parks & Recreation
INFORMATION:	(609) 625-8219
WEB SITE:	www.aclink.org/ parks
OPEN:	April 1–November 1
SITES:	8
EACH SITE HAS:	Picnic table, fire ring
ASSIGNMENT:	At Lake Lenape office
REGISTRATION:	At Lake Lenape office
FACILITIES:	Portable toilet
PARKING:	At site, maximum 2 vehicles
FEE:	$12/night plus $5 administrative fee; pay by check or money order
ELEVATION:	25 feet
RESTRICTIONS:	**Pets:** Prohibited **Fires:** In fire rings by permit ; subject to restrictions **Alcohol:** Prohibited **Vehicles:** No RVs; pop-up campers are allowed **Other:** No wood collecting; 14-night maximum stay; must be at least 21 years of age

ers and wheelchair users. Bicycles, motorized vehicles, and loud noises are prohibited.

Swamp Trail Boardwalk, a six-foot-wide thoroughfare, winds through wetlands and wildlife habitats. It passes deserted building remains from when the Bethlehem Loading Company maintained rail tracks in the area. The Bethlehem Loading Company was one of four munitions production factories that were opened in New Jersey during World War I. All of the steel and iron, including the railroad tracks, were removed and used during World War II. Thousands of people lived and worked in the area in 1918 and 1919. Today little evidence of that time remains.

The boardwalk provides access to nature without damaging the plants underneath the walkway. It also keeps hikers away from ticks and mud. Several more traditional trails, which allow cyclists as well as hikers, wind through the 1,700-acre forest as well. Many of the 15 miles of trails, including the boardwalk, eventually lead to the developed section of Estell Manor, which includes a nature center and a loop road.

The Warren E. Fox Nature Center is the headquarters of the developed section of Estell Manor and is also headquarters for environmental education in Atlantic County. Lectures and meetings are held in its auditorium. Small exhibits detail the area's wildlife activities and explain which trees live within the park. Most popular are the live indigenous animals and carnivorous plants kept in the nature center. Visitors can examine frogs, lizards, turtles, and snails up close.

Fox Nature Center is also home to the Estell Manor bicycle-lending program. Visitors can borrow bikes and helmets at no charge. Also available are volleyballs, Frisbees, softball gear, jump ropes, horseshoes, and soccer balls. All gear must be borrowed and returned during nature center hours (8 a.m.–4 p.m.).

A 2-mile exercise trail begins behind the nature center. The exercise trail parallels the 2.2-mile loop road that passes forest, trails, and picnic areas. The loop also passes the Atlantic County Veteran's Cemetery, which is located within the park.

Visitors will find historic Estellville Glassworks along the loop road, just before the Veteran's Cemetery.

MAP

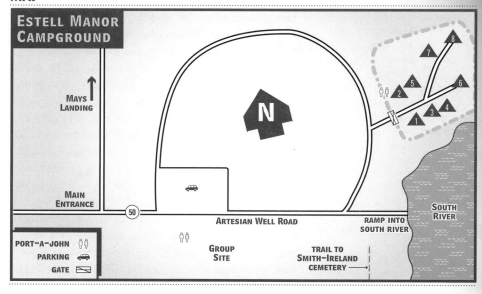

ESTELL MANOR
CAMPGROUND

MAYS
LANDING

N

MAIN
ENTRANCE

50

SOUTH
RIVER

ARTESIAN WELL ROAD

RAMP INTO
SOUTH RIVER

PORT-A-JOHN

PARKING

GATE

GROUP
SITE

TRAIL TO
SMITH-IRELAND
CEMETERY ⟶

Estellville Glassworks operated as a glass-making factory from 1825 to 1877. The three large aboveground buildings that stand today were the melting furnace, the pot house (used for raw material storage), and the flattening house (used in windowpane production). The other partially standing surface buildings are simple and small. They were houses for the workers. The remaining two sites are completely below ground. One was a building used for glass cutting, while the lime shed was used for raw materials storage.

Several picnic tables and pavilions line the road. Picnic Area #2 is near the floating dock on Stephen's Creek. Fishing is permitted from the floating dock, as well as in the South River near the campground. Kayaks and canoes are permitted on Stephen's Creek, but you must carry them in.

However, campers need not make the trip to Stephen's Creek for boating. They can boat on the South River, remaining completely hidden away in the pocket wilderness that makes up the rural camping area at Estell Manor.

GETTING THERE

Follow the Lake Lenape directions (p. 125) to register. Otherwise, from Atlantic City Expressway, take Exit 12E onto County Road 575 South. After 0.3 miles, turn right onto US 40 West. The road turns and winds. After about 4.5 miles, turn left onto NJ 50. The entrance is 1.5 miles down on the left.

ATLANTIC COUNTY PARK AT LAKE LENAPE

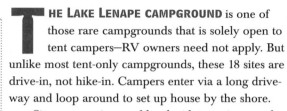

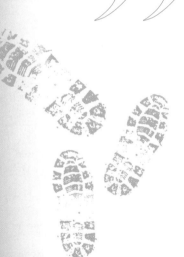

> *This lakeside camp-ground is solely open to tenters; RV owners need not apply.*

THE **LAKE LENAPE CAMPGROUND** is one of those rare campgrounds that is solely open to tent campers—RV owners need not apply. But unlike most tent-only campgrounds, these 18 sites are drive-in, not hike-in. Campers enter via a long drive-way and loop around to set up house by the shore.

Sites are spacious and level with towering woods offering plenty of shade. There's almost no understory, which means no privacy barriers between sites. Campers don't have much privacy from each other, but at least the access road is not a thoroughfare. Only campers use the dead-end drive. Several campsites are located on Lake Lenape itself; sites 7–13 are particularly scenic. Site 18 is exceptionally secluded from the other campsites but unfortunately is located on a 2-mile-long road that leads to a boat launch. Portable toilets dot the camping area, but the more high-tech shower and flush-ing toilets are located near the park entrance at the boathouse. The boathouse is also home to the Atlantic County Rowing Association, a public nonprofit group that promotes rowing in Atlantic County.

Campers can book their site at Lake Lenape one of two ways. They can reserve by phone and complete the application by mail or book in person at the Lake Lenape Reservation Office in the boathouse. Reserve ahead on weekends and also if you expect to arrive late. Permits are not issued after the office closes at 9 p.m. in summer or at 5 p.m. at other times of the camping season. The Lake Lenape Reservation Office also issues permits for Estell Manor camping and for the group sites and ropes course at Camp Acagisca.

The 1,921-acre Atlantic County Park at Lake Lenape is the largest park in the Atlantic County sys-tem. Most of it has been intentionally left wild. It is one of 13 parks acquired through New Jersey State Green Acres funds and a local tax. County citizens

RATINGS

Beauty: ✪ ✪ ✪
Privacy: ✪ ✪
Spaciousness: ✪ ✪ ✪ ✪
Quiet: ✪ ✪ ✪
Security: ✪ ✪
Cleanliness: ✪ ✪

voted the tax into existence in 1990, expressly for the purpose of acquiring open space, recreational land, and historic sites.

Ten miles of trails wind through Lake Lenape's forests. Guided hikes begin at the boathouse on weekends during summer months. Call ahead for the schedule. Naturalists advise hikers to take standard precautions against ticks. Tuck your pant legs into your socks and use insect repellent. Keep your eyes on the sky as well as the trail, as bald eagles are often seen at Lake Lenape in colder months.

The 344-acre lake is home to several species of fish, including bluegill, chain pickerel, yellow perch, crappie, largemouth bass, and sunfish. Fishing is allowed.

Lake Lenape does not allow boats over 20 feet in length. Nonpowered boats are welcome. Canoes, kayaks, sculls, rowboats, and small sailboats are allowed. Access is from the boat ramp near the reservation office. Boaters are asked to check in prior to launching. The ramp is open 365 days a year, from 7:30 a.m. until 30 minutes after sunset.

Kayak, canoe, and small vessel owners may also travel the scenic Great Egg Harbor River. Boaters must purchase permits for $5 at Lake Lenape Boathouse. Leave one permit in your car, which can be left near the boat launch, 250 yards north of campsite 18. Display the other permit in your pick-up vehicle. Boats can also be launched from Camp Acagisca. Canoes can be rented near the park. Parts of Great Egg Harbor River can be difficult and wild; rowers should research routes in advance.

Visitors with motorboats must pay $5 for a yearly permit. Low-powered boats—those with electric motors up to 9.9 horsepower—must be registered. Operators should carry a boat registration card and operator's license. High-powered boats are also allowed on Lake Lenape, but only six boats are permitted on the lake at a time. Ten-horsepower-plus boats must adhere to the same rules as low-powered boats and must also show proof that vessels carry $500,000 worth of liability insurance. The insurance certificate must name Atlantic County as the certificate holder. Call ahead for

KEY INFORMATION

ADDRESS:	Atlantic County Park at Lake Lenape 6303 Harding Highway Mays Landing, NJ 08234
OPERATED BY:	Atlantic County Parks & Recreation
INFORMATION:	(609) 625-8219
WEB SITE:	www.aclink.org/parks
OPEN:	April 1–November 1
SITES:	18
EACH SITE HAS:	Picnic table, fire ring, trash can
ASSIGNMENT:	At office
REGISTRATION:	At office
FACILITIES:	Portable and flush toilets, pay phones, and showers at boathouse
PARKING:	At site, 2-vehicle limit
FEE:	$12, plus $5 administrative fee; pay by check or money order
ELEVATION:	25 feet
RESTRICTIONS:	**Pets:** Prohibited **Fires:** In fire rings by permit **Alcohol:** Prohibited **Vehicles:** No RVs; pop-up campers are allowed **Other:** Must be at least 21 to register; no wood collecting; 14-night limit; check in before 9 p.m.; no swimming from sites

MAP

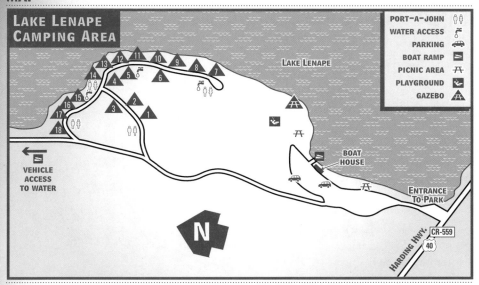

GETTING THERE

From the Atlantic City Expressway, take Exit 12E onto County Road 575 South. After 0.3 miles, turn right onto US 40 West. The road turns and winds. US 40 becomes Harding Highway. The park entrance is on the right after 5.6 miles.

specific details. All boats must possess legal safety equipment.

The Lake Lenape gazebo can be rented for parties, weddings, and other events. It is on the lake next to the playground. Parents must be present when children use the playground, and wet equipment may not be used.

Eight miles northeast of Lake Lenape is 11-acre Weymouth Park. This is a popular takeout spot for canoeists and is also the site of the ruins of Weymouth Forge. Weymouth Forge produced iron for about 60 years during the 1800s. At its height, the tract contained the furnace, 20 houses for workers, a forge, gristmill, church, sawmill, store, barn, blacksmith shop, wheelwright, and owner's mansion. The forge was destroyed in 1862, but its usefulness had already ceased when Pennsylvania coal-powered forges took over.

Some of the forge property was purchased with money from county funds, as was Atlantic County Park at Lake Lenape. The county's dedication to preserving outdoors space is obvious from the excellent upkeep at Lake Lenape and Estell Manor, as is its dedication to tent camping, apparent in the two non-RV campgrounds found in Atlantic County.

BELLEPLAIN STATE FOREST MEISLE FIELD AND CCC CAMP

UNASSUMING AND MODEST when compared to their private campground cousins that pervade the nearby Cape May peninsula, the campgrounds of Belleplain State Forest offer respite from the Shore's dense RV lifestyle. Belleplain, with its 20,000 acres, is not the southernmost of New Jersey's state parks, but it does contain the three southernmost public campgrounds. It's the closest tent campers can get to Cape May without sacrificing their wilderness experience for more organized, close-knit fun. Belleplain is located within the Pinelands National Reserve, a unique ecosystem also known as the Pine Barrens.

Belleplain's centerpiece, 26-acre Lake Nummy, was the Meisle family's cranberry bog before 1933 when the Civilian Conservation Corps Reforestation Relief Act transformed it. Three separate camps were set up, and the CCC got to work digging and constructing. Lake Nummy was then called Meisle Lake and was later renamed after a Lenni Lenape Native American chief.

Meisle Field and CCC Camp are two adjacent campgrounds located at the southern end of Lake Nummy. They are both large loops bisected by roads that create smaller loops. Meisle Field features 14 cabins and five yurts in addition to 49 basic sites. Trailers and tenters are welcome in Meisle Field, but tent campers will want to head to the back of Meisle Field or to CCC Campground for more privacy. Owners of larger RVs will also want to go to the CCC Camp as there are several large, open sites located along its three roads. Both Meisle Field and CCC Camp have modern bathhouses that feature flushing toilets, hot showers, and laundry facilities.

Eagle Fitness Trail, accessed from a dirt track located between Meisle Field and CCC Camp, is a mile-long self-guided fitness loop that features ten exercise stations. After warming up, hikers can tackle a

> *It's the closest tenters can get to Cape May without sacrificing their wilderness experience.*

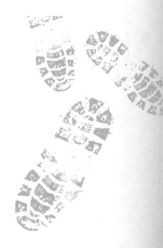

RATINGS

Beauty: ✩ ✩ ✩ ✩
Privacy: ✩ ✩ ✩
Spaciousness: ✩ ✩ ✩ ✩
Quiet: ✩ ✩ ✩
Security: ✩ ✩ ✩
Cleanliness: ✩ ✩ ✩

ADDRESS:	Belleplain State Forest County Route 550 Woodbine, NJ 08270
OPERATED BY:	State Park Service
INFORMATION:	(609) 861-2404
WEB SITE:	www.njparksand forests.org
OPEN:	Meisle, year-round; CCC, April 1– October 31
SITES:	85
EACH SITE HAS:	Picnic table, fire ring
ASSIGNMENT:	Choose from available sites
REGISTRATION:	On arrival or reserve minimum 2 nights
FACILITIES:	Water, flush toilets, showers, laundry
PARKING:	At site, 2-vehicle limit
FEE:	$15
ELEVATION:	35 feet
RESTRICTIONS:	Pets: Prohibited Fires: In fire rings Alcohol: Prohibited Vehicles: No limit Other: Quiet hours 10 p.m.–6 a.m.; 14-night, 6-person, 2-tent limit

long trail such as the 7.16-mile East Creek Trail, or they can just head to Lake Nummy and do a little fishing.

Fishing is also allowed at East Creek Pond, Holly Lake, and Cedar Lake. Pickerel, perch, catfish, and sunfish have been caught in Lake Nummy, while East Creek Pond is also home to largemouth bass. The floating dock on Lake Nummy, near the CCC-built Interpretive Center (once park headquarters), is used for launching small boats and canoes. There is also a boat ramp on the western shore of East Creek Pond. Gas-powered boats may not be used in Belleplain State Forest. Visitors may rent canoes and paddleboats from the floating dock and the swimming area. The bathhouse and white sandy beach are described in the North Shore Campground entry on page 129.

Belleplain State Forest is a great base from which to explore the Victorian seaside resort city of Cape May. It's a 30-mile drive from the campground to the town, but it makes for a pleasant day trip. 2.3-square-mile Cape May is a living-history landmark, a town of restored Victorian homes. Once you have strolled the streets and marveled at the architecture, head over to Cape May Point State Park. Its 235 acres are for day use only, so camping is not allowed.

Cape May Lighthouse is a good place to start your tour of the park. For $5, visitors can climb the 199 steps for a panoramic view of the surrounding peninsula. Back down on earth, during low tide you can see a World War II bunker that was built when the area was a military base. Cape May Point also features a 153-acre natural area, and 4 miles of trails wind through the park so visitors can view regional flora and fauna. But most nature lovers come to Cape May to see one thing—birds.

Cape May is located on a major migratory bird route. The New Jersey Audubon Society maintains the Cape May Bird Observatory. It serves as an information hub and resource center for birders and hosts birding workshops and walks throughout the year. Lists of recently spotted rare birds can be found on its Web site, **www.njaudubon.org,** as well as on its recorded bird hotline (609) 898-BIRD. The Society also hosts the annual World Series of Birding. For 24 hours on a May

MAP

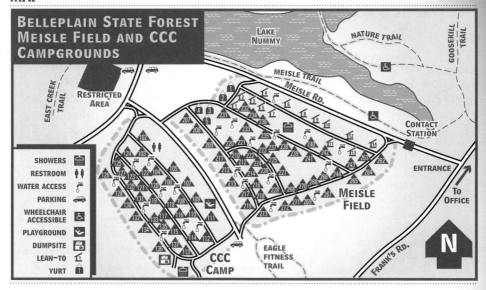

BELLEPLAIN STATE FOREST MEISLE FIELD AND CCC CAMPGROUNDS

SHOWERS
RESTROOM
WATER ACCESS
PARKING
WHEELCHAIR ACCESSIBLE
PLAYGROUND
DUMPSITE
LEAN-TO
YURT

LAKE NUMMY
NATURE TRAIL
GOOSEKILL TRAIL
MEISLE TRAIL
MEISLE RD.
EAST CREEK TRAIL
RESTRICTED AREA
CONTACT STATION
ENTRANCE
To OFFICE
MEISLE FIELD
EAGLE FITNESS TRAIL
CCC CAMP
FRANK'S RD.
N

weekend, teams of birders rush around the state spotting and identifying birds. They must return to Cape May at the end of the day to cross the finish line. Participants have a lot of fun, but the main purpose is not recreation but fund-raising. Sponsors donate money, and one hundred percent of funds raised go to the participants' choice of environmental funds.

Belleplain State Forest is not the most convenient campground to Cape May. More than a dozen campgrounds are located on the Cape May peninsula itself. But most of those sites are RV-oriented, with no privacy or space between sites. They're geared toward shore access, not toward wilderness and nature. At Belleplain State Forest, campers get the best of the lot—natural beauty, seclusion, shore access, and proximity to the Cape May peninsula.

GETTING THERE

From the Garden State Parkway, take Exit 17 to US 9 North. Go 0.5 miles on US 9 North to CR 550. Go left on CR 550 and follow it for 10 miles to the park entrance on the left.

BELLEPLAIN STATE FOREST NORTH SHORE CAMPGROUND

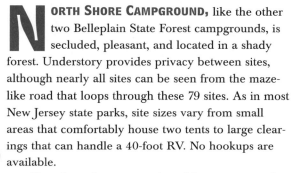

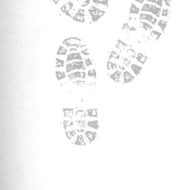

With tranquil campsites and easy access to Cape May peninsula, Belleplain offers the best of both worlds.

NORTH SHORE CAMPGROUND, like the other two Belleplain State Forest campgrounds, is secluded, pleasant, and located in a shady forest. Understory provides privacy between sites, although nearly all sites can be seen from the maze-like road that loops through these 79 sites. As in most New Jersey state parks, site sizes vary from small areas that comfortably house two tents to large clearings that can handle a 40-foot RV. No hookups are available.

Sites along the eastern edge of the campground border Lake Nummy. Most are surrounded by shrubs and bushes, but sites 25 through 27 are open and can provide space for a small group or large family.

Booking ahead might get you a coveted lakeside site because the staff does attempt to satisfy requests, but plenty of scenic nonlakeside spots are available on summer weekdays. Reserve ahead on holidays and weekends.

Belleplain's North Shore Campground is located near 26-acre Lake Nummy's white sandy beach and swim area. The bathhouse, beach, and snack bar are open from Memorial Day weekend through Labor Day. For those who prefer to swim in the sea, the Atlantic Ocean is only 10 miles away.

20,000-acre Belleplain State Forest sprawls across both Cape May and Cumberland County. The park features over 40 miles of trails; some are dedicated solely to hikers while others are multiuse. Fourteen trails offer access to motorized vehicles, but all-terrain vehicles (ATVs) are prohibited throughout the park. Note that several of these motorized trails are backcountry routes and are not passable by regular cars. Some pass through large pools of water or along steep grades. Trucks, snowmobiles, and motorcycles are commonly used on the trails.

RATINGS

Beauty: ✿ ✿ ✿ ✿
Privacy: ✿ ✿ ✿ ✿
Spaciousness: ✿ ✿ ✿ ✿
Quiet: ✿ ✿ ✿ ✿
Security: ✿ ✿ ✿
Cleanliness: ✿ ✿ ✿ ✿

Along with the Eagle Fitness Trail, two trails are dedicated solely to pedestrians. Nature Trail 1 and Nature Trail 2 wind around the northern shore of Lake Nummy and through the nearby forest. These trails feature 32 stations that highlight plants and habitats. Pick up a booklet at the forest office to follow the self-guided route. Hikers should remember that the forest is home to ticks and deer lice. Wear insecticide, long sleeves, trousers, and socks.

The remaining 16 miles of trails are open to hikers, cyclists, horses, and cross-country skiers. Cyclists and hikers must yield to horses. Trails are marked with signs that indicate their designations. All users, regardless of their chosen method for traversing the trails, will enjoy the shade of tall cedar, pine, holly, and laurel trees.

Belleplain State Forest is also a main stop on another sort of trail. It's an information site for the Delsea Region of the New Jersey Coastal Heritage Trail Route, a 300-mile-long auto tour.

The New Jersey Coastal Heritage Trail Route begins where many people first enter New Jersey, near the Delaware Memorial Bridge at the southwestern tip of the state. The route hugs the coast all the way to Cape May in the east, and then follows the Jersey Shore north to Raritan Bay, ending just before the New York City metropolitan area begins. It's a cooperative project involving the National Park Service and New Jersey. The route was established in 1988 and features the five categorical themes of maritime history, coastal habitats, wildlife migration, relaxation and inspiration, and historic settlements. The last two categories are still under development.

Pick up a brochure for the Delsea Region at the forest office, and you can drive from the Delaware Memorial Bridge to Cape May Court House, stopping at designated sites en route. Highlights include wildlife management areas, wetlands, and the Greenwich Tea Burning Monument. In 1774, young men dressed as Native Americans and burned East India tea. This was after the famous Boston Tea Party but prior to the start of the Revolutionary War.

KEY INFORMATION

ADDRESS:	Belleplain State Forest County Route 550 Woodbine, NJ 08270
OPERATED BY:	State Park Service
INFORMATION:	(609) 861-2404
WEB SITE:	www.njparksand forests.org
OPEN:	April 1–October 31
SITES:	79
EACH SITE HAS:	Picnic table, fire ring
ASSIGNMENT:	Choose from available sites
REGISTRATION:	On arrival or reserve minimum 2 nights
FACILITIES:	Water, flush toilets, showers, laundry
PARKING:	At site, 2-vehicle limit
FEE:	$15
ELEVATION:	30 feet
RESTRICTIONS:	Pets: Prohibited Fires: In fire rings only Alcohol: Prohibited Vehicles: No limit Other: Quiet hours 10 p.m.–6 a.m.; 14-night, 6-person, 2-tent limit

MAP

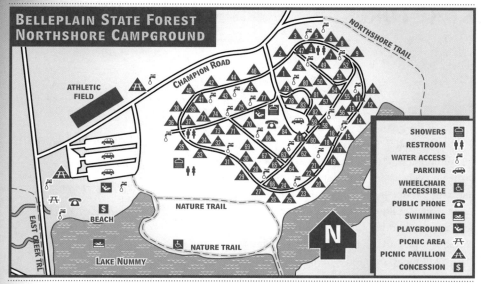

BELLEPLAIN STATE FOREST NORTHSHORE CAMPGROUND

NORTHSHORE TRAIL

CHAMPION ROAD

ATHLETIC FIELD

NATURE TRAIL

NATURE TRAIL

BEACH

LAKE NUMMY

EAST CREEK TRL

SHOWERS	
RESTROOM	
WATER ACCESS	
PARKING	
WHEELCHAIR ACCESSIBLE	
PUBLIC PHONE	
SWIMMING	
PLAYGROUND	
PICNIC AREA	
PICNIC PAVILLION	
CONCESSION	

GETTING THERE

From the Garden State Parkway, take Exit 17 to US 9 North. Go 0.5 miles on US 9 North to CR 550. Go left on CR 550 and follow it for 10 miles to the park entrance on the left.

Another notable feature of the Delsea Region is the annual horseshoe crab spawning at Heislerville Wildlife Management Area. Horseshoe crabs lay eggs on the beach in May, which in turn attracts thousands of migratory shorebirds. Horseshoe crabs and migratory birds can also be observed at East Point Lighthouse. In early fall, you can observe migrating monarch butterflies at East Point Lighthouse.

A bald eagle's nest can be seen at Stow Creek Viewing Area, and bald eagles have also shown up at Heislerville Wildlife Management Area. Other points of interest include post–Civil War Fort Mott and Hancock House Historic Site. The latter was the Revolutionary War massacre site where 30 sleeping colonial militiamen were killed by a British force.

Belleplain State Forest offers the best of both worlds to campers and nature lovers, with its tranquil woodland campsites and easy access to the attractions of the Cape May peninsula. Couples, families, and solo campers will all enjoy the recreational offerings of the park.

BRENDAN T. BYRNE STATE FOREST

THE CLEAN SCENT OF PINE permeates the air at Brendan T. Byrne State Forest campground, reminding visitors that they are in the 1.1 million-acre Pinelands National Reserve, a unique protected ecosystem. Eighty-two wooded sites on three flat, sandy loops make up this northernmost Pineland campground. Like all state campgrounds in New Jersey, there are no RV hookups, although there is a sanitation dump. Yurts sit permanently on sites 14, 15, and 16, providing accommodation for campers who do not own tents. Three cabins, located near Pakim Pond, are also available. Cabin tenants share the campground showers in the two modern bathhouses, but cabins do feature en suite toilets and sinks.

Shrubbery between sites gives the illusion of privacy, but the understory and surrounding forest is less dense than in northern and southwestern Jersey. This is mostly due to environmental differences in spite of the region's history. The forest was clear-cut by Lebanon Glass Works between 1851 and 1867, but you can't tell from today's preponderance of tall trees. The Civilian Conservation Corps replanted the area during the Great Depression.

Lebanon Glass Works employed about 150 men in its heyday, and a small town grew up to support them. The availability of sand and wood for the furnaces provided the ideal situation for the manufacturers of glass for windows and bottles. The glass factory thrived until the forest was depleted. Once the wood ran out, the town was abandoned. The remains of the town can be seen on trails in the form of stone or brick structures and large depressions.

The buildings of Whitesbog Village, a turn-of-the-century berry production town at the northern end of the park, fared better. While the workers' homes were bulldozed in the early 1970s, the central village area is

> *These northernmost Pine Barrens sites are located near old cranberry bogs.*

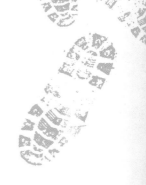

RATINGS

Beauty: ✪ ✪ ✪ ✪
Privacy: ✪ ✪ ✪
Spaciousness: ✪ ✪ ✪
Quiet: ✪ ✪ ✪ ✪
Security: ✪ ✪ ✪
Cleanliness: ✪ ✪ ✪

KEY INFORMATION

ADDRESS: Brendan T. Byrne State Forest
NJ Routes 70 and 72
New Lisbon, NJ 08064

OPERATED BY: State Park Service

INFORMATION: (609) 726-1191

WEB SITE: www.njparksand forests.org

OPEN: Year-round

SITES: 82

EACH SITE HAS: Picnic table, fire ring

ASSIGNMENT: Choose from available sites

REGISTRATION: On arrival or reserve minimum 2 nights

FACILITIES: Water, flush toilets, showers, laundry

PARKING: At site, maximum 2 vehicles

FEE: $15

ELEVATION: 50 feet

RESTRICTIONS: Pets: Prohibited
Fires: In fire rings only
Alcohol: Prohibited
Vehicles: No limit
Other: Quiet hours 10 p.m.–6 a.m.; 14-night, 6-person, 2-tent limit

still standing, and much of it has been restored. Whites-bog was the center for New Jersey cranberry production as well as the first place where blueberries were successfully cultivated. It fell out of use after the Industrial Revolution, when its farming methods became obsolete. Today, New Jersey ranks third in the nation in cranberry production. Some cranberry bogs in the forest are still active. Whitesbog Village is open daily.

More than 25 miles of marked trails crisscross 34,725-acre Brendan T. Byrne State Forest, including 10 miles of the 50-mile Batona Trail. This wilderness hiking trail cuts across Wharton State Forest and Bass River State Forest in addition to Byrne, allowing hikers to traverse the Pinelands (locally called the Pine Barrens). The pink-blazed path is mostly level, with a few small hills and some wet areas. Hikers may camp only at designated campgrounds. No horses or mountain bikes are permitted on Batona Trail.

Mount Misery Trail, an 8.5-mile loop from Mount Misery to Pakim Pond, does allow mountain bikes. So does the 10.8-mile Bike Trail and 2.7-mile Cranberry Trail. Wheelchairs can also be used on the Cranberry Trail, which is paved and open. Horses are permitted on all sand and gravel roads within the forest. In winter, some trails are used by cross-country skiers. Future trails are being planned with multiuse needs under consideration, and all trails are marked with signs that designate their use and accessibility.

Three of the trails—Cranberry, Mount Misery, and Batona—cut across the Cedar Swamp Natural Area, a 735-acre Pine Barrens in miniature. Most of the trees of the Pinelands are represented, including upland pine-oak, oak-pine forest, pitch pine lowland forest, Atlantic white cedar swamp, and swamp pink. The area supports two New Jersey endangered lilies and a similarly endangered rush. Hikers, campers, and other recreational users are reminded that ticks and biting deer-fleas populate the area. Ticks can carry Lyme disease. Take precautions.

Motorized vehicles are allowed on over 50 miles of unmarked gravel and sand roads. Acceptable vehicles include four-wheel-drive autos, motorcycles, and snowmobiles. The potential of becoming bogged down

MAP

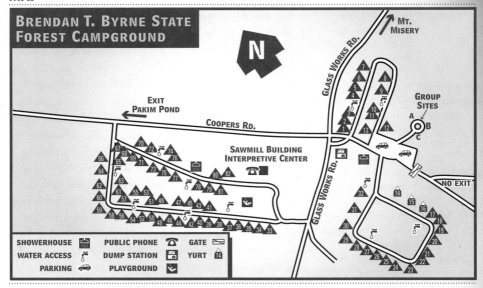

BRENDAN T. BYRNE STATE FOREST CAMPGROUND

MT. MISERY

GLASS WORKS RD.

EXIT
PAKIM POND

COOPERS RD.

GROUP SITES
A
B
C

SAWMILL BUILDING
INTERPRETIVE CENTER

GLASS WORKS RD.

NO EXIT

SHOWERHOUSE		PUBLIC PHONE		GATE	
WATER ACCESS		DUMP STATION		YURT	14
PARKING		PLAYGROUND			

in sand or water on backcountry roads does exist, so motorists should not travel alone and should be prepared. All-terrain vehicles and unlicensed vehicles are prohibited.

Swimming in five-acre Pakim Pond is no longer allowed, but visitors may fish and canoe here, as well as in forest streams.

Brendan T. Byrne State Forest was named Lebanon State Forest until it was renamed in honor of a former governor in 2002. Byrne was the New Jersey governor during most of the 1970s, a tumultuous time in New Jersey history. The forest is referred to as Lebanon State Forest in older publications, but even some new references still use the older name. Either way, the campground in this state forest is worth a stop.

GETTING THERE

From the NJ Turnpike, take Exit 7. Follow US 206 south to NJ 38 east. Turn left onto NJ 38. At the second traffic light, turn right onto Magnolia Road (CR 644). Follow Magnolia Road to Four-Mile Circle. From the circle take NJ 70 east for 1 mile to the forest entrance sign on the right.

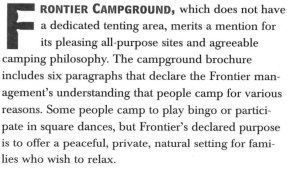

FRONTIER CAMPGROUND

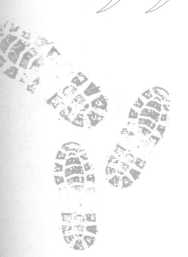

> *Pleasant, wooded sites near the shore are available to all, not just tent campers.*

FRONTIER CAMPGROUND, which does not have a dedicated tenting area, merits a mention for its pleasing all-purpose sites and agreeable camping philosophy. The campground brochure includes six paragraphs that declare the Frontier management's understanding that people camp for various reasons. Some people camp to play bingo or participate in square dances, but Frontier's declared purpose is to offer a peaceful, private, natural setting for families who wish to relax.

RV and tent campers both get the same treatment. Most people associate tent camping with privacy and shady, natural settings. RV campers will be happy to know that they will not be stuck out in a sunny parking lot at Frontier. No, they are given trees and private clearings along with their canvas-covered friends.

This does not mean Frontier is as rustic or secluded as a state park. Those seeking a forest with miles of hiking trails or a park that is a destination unto itself should continue driving to Belleplain State Forest. But for those seeking pleasant, wooded sites along with access to the beach and recreation rooms for the kids, Frontier is the best local option.

Many sites on the 50 acres have privacy barriers, such as hedges and undergrowth. Hardwoods tower over most sites, and each is spacious and clean. The central bathhouse receives frequent cleanings. Sites easily are on par with municipal and county park sites in New Jersey. Note that even though this is a private campground, both pets and alcohol are prohibited.

You won't find a pool at Frontier, but visitors can go fishing and crabbing right by the entrance. For novice campers, the campground features "treehouses" (cabins built on stilts), which come equipped with utensils, linens, and basic furniture. For the kids, there is a

RATINGS

Beauty: ✿ ✿ ✿
Privacy: ✿ ✿ ✿
Spaciousness: ✿ ✿ ✿
Quiet: ✿ ✿ ✿
Security: ✿ ✿ ✿ ✿
Cleanliness: ✿ ✿ ✿ ✿

game room. For the sports-minded, there are ball courts and a playing field.

The famous Jersey Shore is a quick ten-minute drive away. Head northeast to go to Ocean City, with its 2.5-mile boardwalk and amusement pier. Go southeast to reach Sea Isle City, but there is no boardwalk at Sea Isle City. It was destroyed by a storm in 1962 and was replaced by a 1.5-mile blacktop. In between the two cities is Corson's Inlet State Park.

Corson's Inlet State Park is a 350-acre protected coastline area devoted to migratory birds, marine life, and waterfowl. Visitors can view undeveloped beach and waterfront, particularly in the 98-acre Strathmere Natural Area. The park features a free boat ramp, three hiking trails, fishing, crabbing, and interpretive tours. Guided beach walks are scheduled during summer months. Swimming is not allowed at Corson's Inlet, but sunbathing and bird-watching are not only allowed but very popular.

Ten minutes of driving south along Ocean Drive will take you to the Wetlands Institute in Stone Harbor. It's a 34-acre environmental education facility dedicated to the preservation of 6,000 acres of coastal ecosystem. Interpretive programs and hands-on exhibits for children and adults are offered at the center daily. The Wetlands Institute and Corson's Inlet State Park are both points-of-interest on the 300-mile New Jersey Coastal Heritage Trail Route, an auto route that follows the coast from the Delaware Bridge to Perth Amboy. Slightly farther afield from Frontier are the casinos of Atlantic City to the north and the Victorian homes of Cape May to the south. Drive straight up Ocean Drive from Ocean City to enjoy a scenic coastal ride to Atlantic City.

Below Wetlands Institute in North Wildwood is the Hereford Inlet Lighthouse. Built in 1874 and listed on state and national historic registers, the lighthouse is still active and looks more like a Victorian home than a working lighthouse. Tours are available.

Hiking enthusiasts should head to 20,000-acre Belleplain State Forest. Over 40 miles of trails traverse the park. Fourteen of those trails are open to motor

KEY INFORMATION

ADDRESS:	Frontier Campground 84 Tyler Road Ocean View, NJ 08230
OPERATED BY:	Private
INFORMATION:	(609) 390-3649
WEB SITE:	www.frontiercamp ground.com
OPEN:	Mid-April– mid-October
SITES:	9 tent; 196 mixed use
EACH SITE HAS:	Picnic table, fire ring
ASSIGNMENT:	Choose from available sites
REGISTRATION:	On arrival; reservations accepted; 3-day minimum on holidays
FACILITIES:	Water, flush toilets, showers, laundry, store, pay phone
PARKING:	At site
FEE:	$25
ELEVATION:	10 feet
RESTRICTIONS:	**Pets:** Prohibited **Fires:** In fire ring **Alcohol:** Prohibited **Vehicles:** Up to 40 feet **Other:** Quiet hours 11 p.m.–8 a.m.; no woodcutting or collecting; must cover picnic table with tablecloth; use recycling containers; no nails in trees

MAP

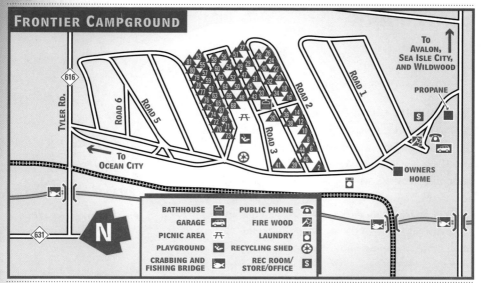

FRONTIER CAMPGROUND

To AVALON, SEA ISLE CITY, AND WILDWOOD

PROPANE

616

TYLER RD.

ROAD 6

ROAD 5

ROAD 4

ROAD 3

ROAD 2

ROAD 1

To OCEAN CITY

OWNERS HOME

631

N

BATHHOUSE		PUBLIC PHONE	
GARAGE		FIRE WOOD	
PICNIC AREA		LAUNDRY	
PLAYGROUND		RECYCLING SHED	
CRABBING AND FISHING BRIDGE		REC ROOM/ STORE/OFFICE	

GETTING THERE

From the Garden State Parkway, take Exit 25. Turn right onto County Road 623 and then left onto CR 631. After 2.8 miles, turn left onto Tyler Road. Follow it for 2 miles to the campground entrance.

vehicles, and 16 miles of trails are designated multiuse. Nature Trails 1 and 2 along with the 1-mile Eagle Fitness Trail are for pedestrians only. The fitness trail features ten exercise stations, while the nature trails include self-guided routes past habitats and plant species. Belleplain's Lake Nummy has a bathhouse and swim area for relaxation after a long day of hiking.

Frontier Campground may not separate tents from RVs, but it does not have to. All sites are equal here, with each being of a high standard normally not seen at RV sites. The location is near the shore, where most campgrounds pack RVs in so densely you would mistake camping for urban living. Peaceful Frontier feels rural without sacrificing convenience.

PARVIN STATE PARK

HUMBLY LOCATED in southwestern Jersey, near no major tourist attractions and no main high-ways, Jaggers Point Campground at Parvin State Park is a destination unto itself. You're not likely to stumble across it while going about your daily business in the Garden State.

But Parvin State Park is well worth a detour. Its campground is one of the nicest in the region. Six small loops are home to 56 sites, giving campers a choice between secluded wooded sites and larger open sites. All are shaded by tall hardwood trees.

Sites 10, 11, and 13 are highly prized due to their lakeside location; book ahead or go midweek to score the waterfront real estate. The camp playground is located next to site 10, so campers lucky enough to stay there may encounter a few young trespassers. There are no trailer hookups, as in all New Jersey State Park Service campgrounds, but RVs are welcome on the larger, open sites. Groups camp separately on a designated island. Additionally, 18 cabins are available for rent from April 1 to October 31.

The cabins and campground, along with Parvin Lake's beach complex and parking lot, were built between 1933 and 1941 by the Civilian Conservation Corps. The CCC, created and deployed as part of FDR's New Deal, built the infrastructure for several of New Jersey's state parks. At Parvin Camp, they dug out and dammed Thundergust Lake, the smaller 14-acre sister to 108-acre Parvin Lake. In 1943, the camp was used as a summer camp for children of displaced Japanese Americans. A year later, it became a POW camp for German prisoners. In 1952, it briefly housed refugees from the Kalmyck Republic, a Caspian Sea state that was abolished by Stalin. The refugees went on to settle in central New Jersey or Philadelphia; Parvin returned to its intended purpose

> *One of the nicest cam grounds in the region, Parvin State Park is well worth a detour.*

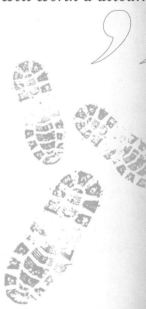

RATINGS

Beauty: ✩ ✩ ✩ ✩
Privacy: ✩ ✩ ✩
Spaciousness: ✩ ✩ ✩ ✩
Quiet: ✩ ✩ ✩ ✩
Security: ✩ ✩ ✩ ✩
Cleanliness: ✩ ✩ ✩ ✩

ADDRESS: Parvin State Park
701 Almond Road
Pittsgrove, NJ 08318

OPERATED BY: State Park Service

INFORMATION: (856) 358-8616

WEB SITE: www.njparksand
forests.org

OPEN: Year-round

SITES: 56

EACH SITE HAS: Picnic table, fire
ring, lantern hooks

ASSIGNMENT: Choose from
available sites

REGISTRATION: On arrival or
reserve minimum 2
nights

FACILITIES: Water, flush toilets,
showers, laundry

PARKING: At site, 2-vehicle
limit

FEE: $15

ELEVATION: 80 feet

RESTRICTIONS: Pets: Prohibited
Fires: In fire rings
only
Alcohol: Prohibited
Vehicles: No limit
Other: Quiet hours
10 p.m.–6 a.m.; 14-
night, 6-person, 2-
tent limit

of providing nature access and recreation to the public.

Parvin Lake features a campground boat ramp exclusively for campers. Cabins have their own boat ramps as well, but the public boat launch is at Fisherman's Landing on the east side of the lake, off Parvin Mill Road. Visitors can rent canoes at Parvin Grove, near the swimming beach, on the north side of the lake. Electrical powered boats are also allowed on both lakes, but only canoeists and people-powered boats can row down the stream Muddy Run, from Parvin Lake to the town of Centerton.

Fishing is popular on both lakes and on Muddy Run. Pickerel, catfish, yellow perch, and sunfish live in Parvin State Park's waters, along with trophy bass. Hunting is prohibited.

Swimming is allowed at the lifeguard-protected beach at Parvin Grove, by the park office. A free parking lot is located across County Road 540, but a fee is charged to enter the beach area. Concessionaires offer snacks and beach supplies, and there are picnic areas, playgrounds, and a bathhouse beside the beach.

Parvin has designated 465 of its 1,309 acres as the "Parvin Natural Area," and that land is permanently protected as undeveloped woodlands. You may spot 172 species of birds here, as well as deer, mice, river otters, frogs, salamanders, toads, turtles, and snakes. The state-endangered barred owl and swamp pink live in the park. More than half of Parvin's 15 miles of trails wind through the natural area, under pitch pines and through cedar swamps. Take precautions against ticks. They are common in south Jersey and particularly prevalent in the natural area. Cover up with long sleeves, pants, socks, and hiking boots and apply insecticide regularly while in the area.

Sooner or later, most campers at Parvin State Park must head to Vineland for supplies. It's the nearest city and home to restaurants, gas stations, and supermarkets. But Vineland has some other claims to semifame. It's the original home of Welch's Grape Juice and mason jars. The Statue of Liberty also resides in Vineland. No, not THAT Statue of Liberty (although some argue that Liberty Island is also in Jersey) . . . the

MAP

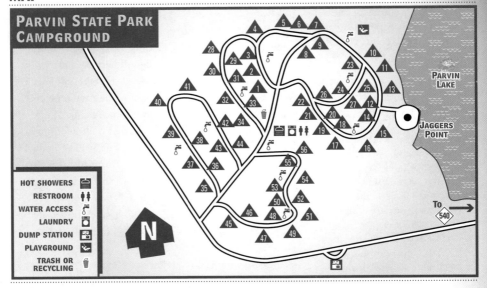

PARVIN STATE PARK CAMPGROUND

HOT SHOWERS
RESTROOM
WATER ACCESS
LAUNDRY
DUMP STATION
PLAYGROUND
TRASH OR RECYCLING

PARVIN LAKE

JAGGERS POINT

To 540

N

concrete Vineland version is 30 feet tall and resides in a private backyard statuary built by local resident George Arbuckel during the Great Depression. The statue is visible from Main Street.

The CCC and Arbuckel were not the only ones busily building during the Depression. Vineland's George Daynor created an 18-spired castle out of junk and old cars. The Palace Depression stood as an income-generating landmark for many years but fell into disrepair before it was finally destroyed in 1969. The Palace of Depression Restoration Association is currently restoring the Palace. So when in Vineland, drive down Mill Road near Landis Avenue and have a look at their progress.

Another attraction potentially worth a detour is the Cowtown Rodeo, some 22 miles northwest of Parvin State Park on US 40 past Sharptown. Saturday night rodeos have occurred there weekly since 1929.

Southwestern New Jersey and Parvin State Park are unique in the state. The crowds teeming along the shore and in the north are not found here, and a hike through Parvin Natural Area will most likely be a solitary, enjoyable affair.

GETTING THERE

From I-295, take Exit 26 to NJ 42 South. Drive 1.3 miles to NJ 55 South. Take NJ 55 South for about 30 miles to Exit 35. Follow the signs to the park on CR 540.

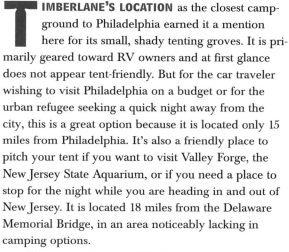

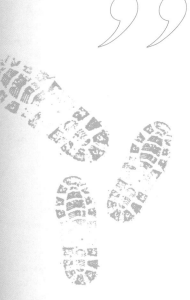

> *The 14 shady tent sites at Timberlane are great for Philadelphia-bound travelers on budgets.*

TIMBERLANE'S LOCATION as the closest campground to Philadelphia earned it a mention here for its small, shady tenting groves. It is primarily geared toward RV owners and at first glance does not appear tent-friendly. But for the car traveler wishing to visit Philadelphia on a budget or for the urban refugee seeking a quick night away from the city, this is a great option because it is located only 15 miles from Philadelphia. It's also a friendly place to pitch your tent if you want to visit Valley Forge, the New Jersey State Aquarium, or if you need a place to stop for the night while you are heading in and out of New Jersey. It is located 18 miles from the Delaware Memorial Bridge, in an area noticeably lacking in camping options.

The crowded, sunny RV sites may appear unwelcoming to rustic tent campers, but there are three small areas dedicated to tenting. One of the areas is highly recommended, and the other two are acceptable as well. The best sites are 48 through 54, positioned across from a central duck pond and isolated from RVs. Sites are spacious, wooded, and perfect for those seeking a pleasant campground for access to Philadelphia as opposed to the usual outdoors experience.

Timberlane's 20 acres include private campground amenities, including ball courts, a playground, a recreation room with games, horseshoes, shuffleboard, a pool, a store, and pond fishing. The restrooms are clean and maintained. Each tent site has a fire ring, and firewood is sold in the store at the entrance.

The location, near the oil refineries along the Delaware River and an industrial park, is not the top destination in New Jersey for outdoors activities. But a true New Jerseyan never assumes that the presence of refineries excludes the presence of parks and lakes. Just 5 miles to the southwest of Timberlane is Gloucester

RATINGS

Beauty: ✿ ✿
Privacy: ✿ ✿
Spaciousness: ✿ ✿
Quiet: ✿ ✿
Security: ✿ ✿ ✿ ✿
Cleanliness: ✿ ✿ ✿

County's Greenwich Lake Park. The 40-acre Greenwich Lake is a renowned trout-stocked fishing lake. Boating is allowed, and picnic facilities and a playground are available.

A 10-mile drive in the opposite direction takes you to 300-acre Washington Lake Park in Sewell. The park features trails, soccer fields, ball fields, an amphitheater, a gazebo, and a skateboard/in-line skating park and roller hockey rink. The main lake is off-limits to fishing, but there is a separate fishing lake. Free summer concerts and movies sometimes are available in the amphitheater. Trails are planned to extend from Washington Lake Park to 60-acre James G. Atkinson Memorial Park, located a few miles away along Mantua Creek in Hurffville.

Seven miles to the northwest of Timberlane Campground, on the Delaware River, is Red Bank Battlefield Park. Although the name may imply otherwise, the Battle of Red Bank was not fought on the Atlantic coast in the town of Red Bank. This Revolutionary War battle was fought at Fort Mercer, located to the north of the 400-acre Red Bank Plantation that is the park's site. Whitall House, the 1748 Georgian mansion that is the park's centerpiece, was used as a hospital after the battle. The house is open for tours, and the grounds, complete with walkways and natural landscaping, are open for walks.

But most campers do not come to Timberlane for the nearby outdoors activities. They come for the access to Philadelphia, home of the Liberty Bell and Independence Hall. They come to wander the narrow streets in the older parts of town, take a side trip to Valley Forge, and to visit a slice of American history. But don't ignore the Jersey side. Ben Franklin allegedly made the first Jersey joke, calling the state a barrel tapped at both ends. Be sure to get both sides of the story by returning to the Garden State after visiting the Benjamin Franklin National Memorial in Philadelphia's Franklin Institute Science Museum.

Back on the Jersey side, don't miss the New Jersey State Aquarium in Camden. The aquarium reopened in May of 2005 after major renovations. It now features a 40-foot walk-through shark tunnel and a faux

KEY INFORMATION

ADDRESS:	Timberlane Campground 117 Timberlane Road Clarksboro, NJ 08020
OPERATED BY:	Private
INFORMATION:	(856) 423-6677
WEB SITE:	www.timberlane campground.com
OPEN:	Year-round
SITES:	14 tent sites; 82 RV sites
EACH SITE HAS:	Picnic table, fire ring
ASSIGNMENT:	Choose from available sites or reserve ahead
REGISTRATION:	On arrival; reservations recommended
FACILITIES:	Water, flush toilets, showers, laundry, store, pay phone
PARKING:	At site
FEE:	2 adults, $24; children age 10 and older, $3
ELEVATION:	30 feet
RESTRICTIONS:	**Pets:** On leash **Fires:** In fire rings subject to restrictions **Alcohol:** Prohibited in pool area; permitted at site **Vehicles:** No limit **Other:** Quiet hours 11 p.m.–7 a.m.

MAP

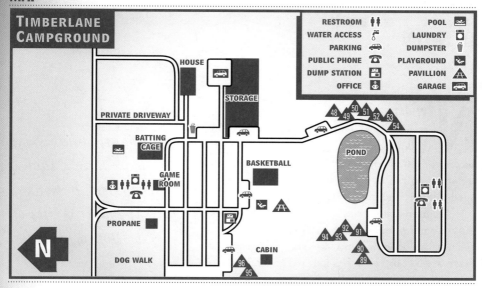

TIMBERLANE CAMPGROUND

RESTROOM	🚻	POOL	🏊
WATER ACCESS		LAUNDRY	
PARKING	🚗	DUMPSTER	🗑
PUBLIC PHONE	☎	PLAYGROUND	
DUMP STATION		PAVILLION	⛺
OFFICE		GARAGE	🚐

HOUSE

STORAGE

PRIVATE DRIVEWAY

BATTING CAGE

BASKETBALL

GAME ROOM

POND

PROPANE

N

DOG WALK

CABIN

GETTING THERE

From I-295 southbound, take Exit 18. Follow County Road 667 south to Friendship Road. Go right one block to Timberlane Road. Turn right to the campground.

West African river complete with hippopotamuses. The battleship New Jersey, now a museum, is permanently anchored nearby.

Timberlane Campground is also the closest campground to the start of the New Jersey Coastal Heritage Trail. Not many people drive the entire 300 miles of this vehicular trail in one trip, but if you want to be a thru-driver, start at the Delaware Memorial Bridge, stopping en route at Fort Mott State Park in Pennsville. It is the Welcome Center for the Delsea Region and the first (or last from the other direction) information center along the route. Fort Mott was built right after the Civil War. Troops were stationed there for many years, but it became obsolete with the advent of modern defenses. Today it is a 104-acre free park with an easy nature trail and picnic facilities.

Most campers ignore the southeastern part of New Jersey due to its lack of campgrounds. But there is no shortage of activities and outdoor opportunities. Stop for a few nights at Timberlane and give this often-neglected part of the state a look.

WHARTON STATE FOREST: ATSION

NEW **JERSEY'S LARGEST** state forest has nine camping areas, with the capacity to hold over a thousand campers, but only 50 sites have access to flushing toilets and hot showers. These sites are at Atsion Family Campsites, the only fully developed campground in Wharton State Forest.

Atsion may not be as remote or secluded as many of Wharton's primitive wilderness areas, but sites are beautifully wooded and private. The campground is easily reached by car. It has four paved loops suitable for small trailers as well as tents, although there are no hookups. Sites along the inner loops are close to the lake and farther from Atsion Road. Nine furnished cabins also sit along Atsion Road and look out over Atsion Lake.

An added bonus of staying at either Atsion Family Campsites or the lakeside cabins is that access to nearby Atsion Recreation Area is included in the nightly fee. Remember to carry your permit for free access. Campers at wilderness sites pay only $1 a person per night to camp, but parking at the recreation area then costs $5 per car on weekdays and $10 on weekends. Walk-ins pay $2. Cars bearing current New Jersey State Park annual passes park for free. Once the parking lot has reached full capacity (300 vehicles), vehicles are asked to wait regardless of permits.

Atsion Recreation Area sits directly across from the campground, on the southern side of Atsion Lake. It's a long walk around the lake, so drive or ride a bicycle. There is a guarded swimming beach, open during the summer (Memorial Day weekend to Labor Day) from 10 a.m. to 6 p.m. It is popular with groups, so go early to avoid the crowds. The bathhouse is in a full-service complex that includes men's and women's changing rooms with showers and flushing toilets, a concessionaire, and a first-aid station.

> *Wharton has space for more than a thousand campers, but only Atsion's 50 sites offer developed facilities.*

RATINGS

Beauty: ✦ ✦ ✦
Privacy: ✦ ✦ ✦
Spaciousness: ✦ ✦ ✦
Quiet: ✦ ✦ ✦
Security: ✦ ✦ ✦
Cleanliness: ✦ ✦ ✦

ADDRESS: Wharton State Forest
Atsion Office
744 US 206
Shamong, NJ 08088

OPERATED BY: State Park Service

INFORMATION: (609) 268-0444

WEB SITE: www.njparksand
forests.org

OPEN: April 1–December
31

SITES: 50

EACH SITE HAS: Picnic table, fire ring

ASSIGNMENT: Choose from
available sites

REGISTRATION: Obtain permit at
Atsion office

FACILITIES: Water, flush toilets,
showers

PARKING: At site, 2-vehicle
limit

FEE: $15

ELEVATION: 40 feet

RESTRICTIONS: Pets: Prohibited
Fires: In fire rings
only
Alcohol: Prohibited
Vehicles: Up to 26
feet
Other: Quiet hours
10 p.m.–6 a.m.; 14-
night, 6-person, 2-
tent limit

The recreation area also features two playgrounds, a playing field, and picnic facilities. Only charcoal fires are permitted in the grills provided. A short nature trail loops around behind the playing field, and you'll find restrooms on either end of the parking lot. Fishing is allowed from the dock and on the lake. Visitors are given trash bags upon entering the recreation area and are reminded to remove all their garbage as Wharton State Forest is a carry-in/carry-out area. Alcohol is not allowed at the campsites, picnic areas, or beach, as in all New Jersey state parks.

A public boat launch is at the western end of the beach in the recreation area. It is ADA accessible and is open 8 a.m. to 4 p.m. from Memorial Day to Labor Day. There is no boat rental concession, but canoes can be rented from several locations. The closest is Adams Canoe Rental on Atsion Road near the campground (call (609) 268-0189). Only electric and unpowered boats are allowed on Atsion Lake. Engines must be under 10 horsepower. The other nearby boat launch is the Mullica River canoe put-in located across US 206 from Atsion Lake.

Today Wharton State Forest sprawls over three counties and features 115,000 wooded acres that reach almost from the Atlantic Ocean to 40 miles shy of Philadelphia. Deer, turkeys, beavers, foxes, bald eagles, river otters, and a huge variety of birds live in the forest. Trails and rivers are popular with hikers, bikers, equestrians, boaters, birders, and other outdoors enthusiasts.

Surprisingly, Wharton State Forest, once inhabited by Leni-Lenape Native Americans, was an industrial area from 1766 to 1867. Naturally occurring bog ore was mined from the swamps during the American Revolution and the War of 1812. Bog ore is formed when organic acids from vegetation combine with clay that is rich with iron. Wharton's many streams and rivers created the ideal processing environment for the bog ore that was turned into bog iron and used for munitions. Later, Wharton was the site of both glassmaking and papermaking operations, as were other parts of the Pinelands.

When Philadelphia financier Joseph Wharton purchased thousands of acres in southern Jersey in 1876,

MAP

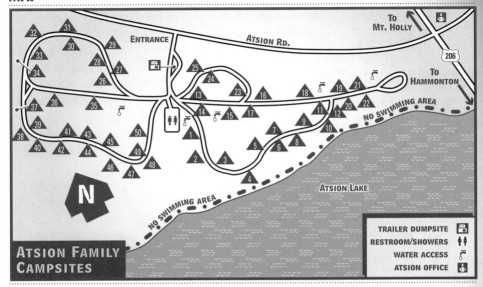

ATSION FAMILY CAMPSITES

TRAILER DUMPSITE	
RESTROOM/SHOWERS	
WATER ACCESS	
ATSION OFFICE	

he had plans to sell the clean groundwater to Philadelphia. New Jersey's government passed a law banning him from doing so. Wharton still appreciated his property and continued to acquire more throughout his life. New Jersey bought the land in the 1950s for access to the same water that Wharton had astutely valued. His accidental preservation and later foresight led to the protection of the heart of the Pine Barrens. Campers can enjoy the scenic clearings at Atsion and throughout Wharton today due to Wharton's purchase.

GETTING THERE

From the New Jersey Turnpike, take Exit 7 to US 206 South. Drive about 28 miles south on US 206 to Atsion Road. The office is at the intersection. Turn right to the campground entrance.

WHARTON STATE FOREST: BATONA CAMP

Quiet, simple Batona Camp sits directly astride the famous Batona Trail.

FAR FROM THE BEATEN PATH sits distant Batona Camp, directly across the road from Carranza Memorial. No sites are demarcated on the ground alongside the unimproved sand road, and fire pits made by past campers are the only indication that campers have stopped here for the night. Two outhouses, a water (potable) pump, and a sign are the developed features here under the pitch pines.

Campers will encounter little auto traffic in the campground, but they may meet a hiker or two. Batona Camp sits in the sand alongside the legendary Batona Trail, a 50-mile mostly flat hiking path that traverses the Pinelands National Reserve. The Batona (or BAck TO NAture Trail) Trail passes through parts of Brendan T. Byrne State Forest and Bass River State Forest as it winds its way across the Pinelands, but more than half of it is located within Wharton State Forest. The trail runs the length of the camping area, meandering right down the middle. Campers should avoid setting up tents squarely on the trail.

For those interested in a shorter Batona Trail hike, the section between Carranza Memorial and Apple Pie Hill is a popular alternative to walking the entire 50 miles. Apple Pie Hill is 3.5 miles north of the camping area, on the Batona Trail just outside the Wharton State Forest border. The hill, at 205 feet, is the highest point in the Pine Barrens (the local name for the Pinelands). Hike to the top of the 60-foot-tall tower for sweeping views of the 1.1 million-acre reserve, which sits above 17 trillion gallons of clean groundwater. On clear days, it is possible to see from the Atlantic Ocean to the Delaware River, with Atlantic City visible to the east and Philadelphia to the west.

The walk back to Carranza Memorial takes you through cedar swamps and under tall hardwoods. Carranza Memorial itself is a tall stone obelisk dedicated

RATINGS

Beauty: ✫ ✫ ✫ ✫
Privacy: ✫ ✫ ✫
Spaciousness: ✫ ✫ ✫ ✫
Quiet: ✫ ✫ ✫ ✫ ✫
Security: ✫ ✫
Cleanliness: ✫ ✫ ✫

to 23-year-old Mexican pilot Captain Emilio Carranza. He crashed here during a thunderstorm in 1928. Sometimes referred to as the Lindbergh of Mexico, he was on the homeward-bound section of a Mexico City-to-New York City goodwill journey. The obelisk was paid for by donations from Mexican schoolchildren. The 3.5-mile Carranza Memorial Loop goes southeast from the monument and is a popular hike. It combines local dirt roads with a section of the Batona Trail.

The Batona Trail is strictly for hikers. Cyclists and horseback riders are prohibited from wandering along the pink-blazed path, although horses are allowed in Batona Camp in designated areas. Dozens of sand and dirt roads crisscross Wharton State Forest and most of those are open to multiple uses. When the Batona Trail merges with dirt roads, those sections are multiuse. The 6.5-mile Sandy Ridge to Pine Crest Trail, which begins 2.5 miles southeast of the campground, is open to all.

Skit Branch, a narrow creek, sits beyond a line of trees at the northern end of Batona Camp. Sit on the shore in the evenings and listen for frog calls.

Batona Camp is occasionally the site for Russ Juelg's "Jersey Devil Hunts." Around a campfire, Juelg tells stories of the Pinelands most famous legendary resident, the perhaps-fictional Jersey Devil. Check **www.pinelandsalliance.org** or call the Pinelands Preservation Alliance at (609) 859-886 for details. The PPA has plenty of other activities on its schedule as well, including orienteering, hikes, and outdoors survival workshops. Orienteering is particularly useful in the Pinelands because much of the landscape is similar, with few distinguishing landmarks.

If hiking to your site at Batona Camp, remember that you are required to obtain a camping permit in advance at either the Atsion or Batsto Wharton State Forest office. This is best scouted out and done by vehicle as both offices are miles away from the camping area. The road from US 206 to Carranza Memorial is paved, but the 0.2-mile driveway into the campground is dirt. Bear in mind that the road becomes much sandier past the camping area and should not be attempted by novices in sedans, particularly while it is raining.

ADDRESS: Wharton State Fore Atsion Office
744 US 206
Shamong, NJ 08088

OPERATED BY: State Park Service

INFORMATION: (609) 268-0444

WEB SITE: www.njparksand forests.org

OPEN: Year-round

SITES: Open area; maximum 150 people

EACH SITE HAS: Picnic table, fire rin

ASSIGNMENT: Choose from available spaces

REGISTRATION: Obtain permit at either Atsion or Batsto office

FACILITIES: Water, vault toilets

PARKING: At site, 2-vehicle limit

FEE: $1 per person

ELEVATION: 70 feet

RESTRICTIONS: Pets: Prohibited
Fires: In fire rings only
Alcohol: Prohibited
Vehicles: Up to 21 feet
Other: Quiet hours 10 p.m.–6 a.m.; 14-night, 6-person, 2-tent limit

MAP

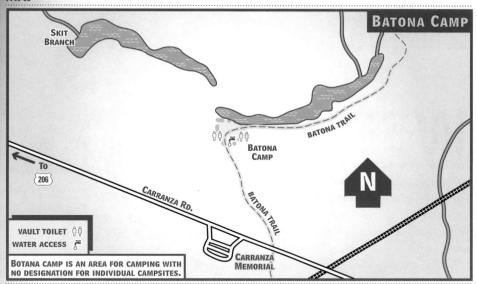

SKIT
BRANCH

BATONA TRAIL

BATONA
CAMP

To
206

CARRANZA RD.

BATONA TRAIL

N

VAULT TOILET
WATER ACCESS

BOTANA CAMP IS AN AREA FOR CAMPING WITH
NO DESIGNATION FOR INDIVIDUAL CAMPSITES.

CARRANZA
MEMORIAL

GETTING THERE

From the New Jersey Turn-pike, take Exit 7 to US 206 South. Drive south for about 20 miles. Veer left onto Carranza Road (CR 648). Drive straight to the Carranza Memorial. The dirt road on the left across from Carranza Memorial leads 0.2 miles to Batona Campground.

Sites at Batona Camp are isolated and beautiful. There is shade and the sound of crickets and wind rustling the pines overhead. If you are a hiker who enjoys inexpensive, quiet, and lovely sites, and you do not require the presence of a bathhouse, Batona Camp is the ideal camping area for you.

WHARTON STATE FOREST: BODINE FIELD

WHARTON STATE FOREST'S easternmost camping area is also its largest. Bodine Field Camp, officially capable of holding up to 250 people, is ideal for large groups. Wharton staff also recommends it for use by equestrian groups. The sandy ground is level and wide-open. The area is sunny, with only some shade. Sites are not designated in this wilderness camping area. Camp anywhere that suits you.

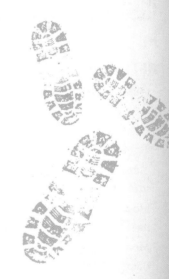

This is Pinelands wilderness camping for those who like to rough it.

When no large groups are present, Bodine Field is great for family or small group camping. It is an inexpensive, sunny, riverside area with good access by both unimproved road and canoe routes. Be cautious when bringing in your car as the sandy roads can get swampy after a rain. Vehicles with four-wheel drive should have no problem.

Like many wilderness camping areas in Wharton State Forest, Bodine Field is popular with canoeists. Beaver Branch Canoe Landing lies just beyond the camp and is the end point on several daily Wading River canoe routes from as nearby as Evans Bridge (two hours) and as far as Speedwell (eight hours). Those who have planned ahead and obtained advance permits from Batsto Visitor Center can stop 20 minutes before Beaver Branch at Bodine Field and set up camp. If possible, leave a vehicle with camping gear at Bodine Field so you can avoid carrying it in your canoe. At least seven canoe liveries serve the area for those who need to rent canoes. The nearest ones include Bel Haven Canoe, Kayak and Tubes in Green Bank (**www.belhavencanoe.com**); Mick's Canoe and Kayak Rental in Jenkins (**www.mickscanoerental. com**); Pine Barrens Canoe and Kayak Rental in Chatsworth (**www.pinebarrenscanoe.com**); and Wading Pines Camping Resort near Godfrey Bridge Campground (**www.wadingpines.com**).

RATINGS

Beauty: ✿ ✿ ✿
Privacy: ✿ ✿ ✿
Spaciousness: ✿ ✿ ✿ ✿
Quiet: ✿ ✿ ✿ ✿
Security: ✿ ✿
Cleanliness: ✿ ✿ ✿

ADDRESS: Wharton State Forest
Batsto Office
4110 Nesco Road
Hammonton, NJ
08037

OPERATED BY: State Park Service

INFORMATION: (609) 561-0024

WEB SITE: www.njparksand
forests.org

OPEN: Year-round

SITES: Open area; maximum 250 people

EACH SITE HAS: Picnic table, fire ring

ASSIGNMENT: Choose from
available spaces

REGISTRATION: Obtain permit at
Batsto office

FACILITIES: Water, vault toilets

PARKING: At site, 2-vehicle
limit.

FEE: $1 per pserson

ELEVATION: 30 feet

RESTRICTIONS: **Pets:** Prohibited
Fires: In fire rings
only
Alcohol: Prohibited
Vehicles: Up to 21
feet
Other: Quiet hours
10 p.m.–6 a.m.; 14-
night, 6-person, 2-
tent limit

Cyclists also have plenty of opportunities for fun in the area surrounding Bodine Field. The popular 17-mile Harrisville Lake to Evans Bridge paved cycling loop begins right above Bodine Field at Harrisville Lake on County Road 679. Head southeast to CR 653 and then go right, following CR 542 to Green Bank. There is a picnic area at Green Bank. Follow CR 563 north to CR 679, which takes you back to your starting point by Harrisville Lake and the Harrisville Ruins. You'll pass through Bass River State Forest as well as Wharton. Some of the roads feature bicycle lanes.

The Pine Barrens River Ramble bike route also passes by Harrisville Lake on its 42-mile loop. A map is available from New Jersey's Department of Transportation as a free download from **www.state.nj.us/njcommuter/html/bikemaps.htm.** The route passes through forests, historical areas, blueberry fields, and cranberry bogs. Standard bicycles are restricted to paved roads, but mountain bikes have the run of the hundreds of sand roads through the Pine Barrens.

The Harrisville Ruins are all that remains of a once-thriving paper mill town. The decaying stone buildings, some of which had three-foot-thick walls, were active in the 1800s. Like many of the nearby industries, the paper industry made use of the surrounding natural resources. Salt marsh grass from the Jersey Shore was brought in and processed using the vast reserves of Pine Barrens water. Canals and mill-races crisscrossed the area. Prior to being a paper mill town, Harrisville was an iron processing facility that made iron into strips, and was the site of a gristmill and two sawmills as early as 1750. Joseph Wharton, the man who eventually acquired most of what is now Wharton State Forest, purchased the property around 1896. The town, which was by then uninhabited, was devastated by fire in 1914.

Once you are done marveling at man-made objects being reclaimed by the forest, take a ride over to the 1,927-acre Oswego River Natural Area for a look at a forest that has been deliberately preserved by mankind. This region, along with the Batsto Natural Area north of Batsto Village, features a variety of pinelands habitats. You'll spot pitch pines, white

MAP

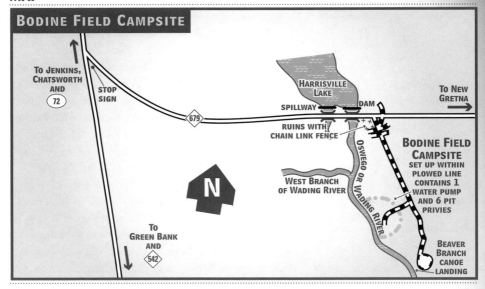

BODINE FIELD CAMPSITE

To Jenkins, Chatsworth and 72

Stop Sign

679

To Green Bank and 542

N

Harrisville Lake

Spillway   Dam

To New Gretna

Ruins with Chain Link Fence

West Branch of Wading River

Oswego or Wading River

BODINE FIELD CAMPSITE
SET UP WITHIN PLOWED LINE
CONTAINS 1 WATER PUMP AND 6 PIT PRIVIES

Beaver Branch Canoe Landing

cedars, southern swamps, and floodplains. You may hear the endangered Pine Barrens treefrog during breeding season (May to June). The treefrog is only an inch and a half long and green, making it difficult to spot. But its nasal honking, often referred to as a "kwonk," is unmistakable.

Swimming is prohibited outside Atsion Recreation Area in Wharton State Forest. Tubing, however, is acceptable, so feel free to launch a tube alongside Bodine Field. There is a small beach at Atsion Recreation Area, but the guarded swimming area at Lake Absegami in Bass River State Forest is closer to Bodine Field.

The Wading River, which meets up with the Oswego River just above Bodine Field, is the most popular river in the Pinelands. It is easy to paddle and passes by cranberries and under pitch pines. And at the end of the west branch sits Bodine Field, an open wilderness camp where you can beach your canoe and sleep under the stars.

GETTING THERE

From the Garden State Parkway, take Exit 52 toward Batsto. Turn right onto CR 654, which will veer left and become Stage Road after 1.4 miles. Veer left onto CR 653 and drive for 1 mile. Turn right onto CR 679. After 5.6 miles, turn right onto CR 563.

WHARTON STATE FOREST: BUTTONWOOD HILL CAMP

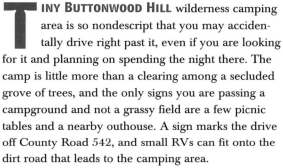

> *Tiny Buttonwood Hill offers inexpensive, primitive camping with good road access and proximity to Batsto Village.*

TINY **BUTTONWOOD HILL** wilderness camping area is so nondescript that you may accidentally drive right past it, even if you are looking for it and planning on spending the night there. The camp is little more than a clearing among a secluded grove of trees, and the only signs you are passing a campground and not a grassy field are a few picnic tables and a nearby outhouse. A sign marks the drive off County Road 542, and small RVs can fit onto the dirt road that leads to the camping area.

Twenty-five people can officially fit into Buttonwood, but on weekdays there's a good chance your party will be the only one in sight. The area is essentially a half circle alongside an unimproved road that becomes increasingly unimproved as it winds deeper into the forest. The road continues through to Bulltown and is definitely for four-wheel-drive vehicles only. Flushing toilets and water are located across CR 542 at Crowley Landing public boat launch. No fees are charged at Crowley Landing, which sits on the Mullica River and features picnic tables and grills in addition to modern restrooms. Motorized boats can be launched here, so don't expect pristine forest conditions. Crowley Landing is within walking distance of Buttonwood Hill, but consider driving so you can return carrying your supply of water.

Crowley Landing stands on the site of what may once have been Crowleytown. During the 1850s and 1860s, a glassworks and small town sat on the site. As with so many industrial sites from that era in the Pine Barrens, Crowleytown faded away and disappeared.

Nearby Batsto Village fared better against the assault of time. For a hundred years, industry thrived at Batsto. First, prior to the American Revolution, Charles Read of Burlington established an iron furnace that was used to process bog ore dug out of the swampy

RATINGS

Beauty: ☆ ☆ ☆
Privacy: ☆ ☆ ☆
Spaciousness: ☆ ☆
Quiet: ☆ ☆ ☆
Security: ☆ ☆
Cleanliness: ☆ ☆ ☆

Pineland grounds. John Cox bought Batsto Iron Works from Read and operated it during the war, providing munitions, artillery fittings, and iron fastenings to the Continental Army. Bog ore occurs naturally when decaying vegetation seeps down to iron-rich clay.

From 1784 to 1876, William Richards and his descendents operated Batsto. First it continued as an iron production facility, manufacturing water pipes and firebacks (cast-iron plates lining the brick wall of fireplaces). Once the iron industry declined, Batsto was a window glass production plant for a decade. After the economic failure of the glassmaking operation, Philadelphia financier Joseph Wharton purchased Batsto as part of his plan to pump the Pine Barrens water to Philadelphia. His scheme was later blocked by New Jersey's government.

During Batsto's industrial heyday, hundreds of people lived and worked in Batsto Village before it fell into disrepair. Today, Batsto Village has been restored. Visitors can wander through 33 historic buildings, including a gristmill, icehouse, wheelwright shop, general store, workers' homes, and a post office. The post office is one of four oldest U.S. post offices currently operating. It was never assigned a zip code, and all stamps are canceled by hand.

When Joseph Wharton took over Batsto, he added new buildings and enlarged the existing mansion in the Italianate style of the era. Except when closed for renovations, 14 rooms of the mansion are open to the public. Seasonal 45-minute guided tours of the mansion and the village are on offer for a small fee during busy summer weekends. Self-guided village tours are available at other times. Visitors must pay a parking fee at Batsto during summer weekends and on holidays.

Located between the village sawmill and the workers' homes on the banks of Batsto Lake is the Annie M. Carter Interpretive Center. The focus of the center's displays is on the ecology of the Pinelands and the impact of humans on the area. Activities include slide and video programs, live animal displays, nature hikes, and discussions. The Interpretive Center has eight canoes available for guided nature trips on Batsto Lake. Several hiking trails of 1- to 3.8-mile lengths

KEY INFORMATION

ADDRESS:	Wharton State Forest Batsto Office 4110 Nesco Road Hammonton, NJ 08037
OPERATED BY:	State Park Service
INFORMATION:	(609) 561-0024
WEB SITE:	www.njparksand forests.org
OPEN:	Year-round
SITES:	Open area; 25-person limit
EACH SITE HAS:	Picnic table, fire ring
ASSIGNMENT:	Choose from available spaces
REGISTRATION:	Obtain permit at Batsto office
FACILITIES:	Water nearby, vault toilets
PARKING:	At site, 2-vehicle limit
FEE:	$1 per person
ELEVATION:	10 feet
RESTRICTIONS:	Pets: Prohibited Fires: In fire rings only Alcohol: Prohibited Vehicles: Up to 21 feet Other: Quiet hours 10 p.m.–6 a.m.; 14-night, 6-person, 2-tent limit

MAP

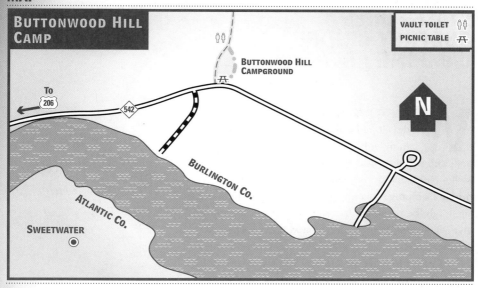

BUTTONWOOD HILL CAMP

VAULT TOILET
PICNIC TABLE

BUTTONWOOD HILL CAMPGROUND

To 206

542

N

BURLINGTON CO.

ATLANTIC CO.

SWEETWATER

GETTING THERE

From the Garden State Parkway, take Exit 52 towards Batsto. Turn right onto CR 654, which becomes Stage Road. Veer left onto CR 653 and drive for 3.2 miles until the road become CR 542. Drive 6.3 miles to Buttonwood Hill entrance on the right.

begin at Batsto and loop through the woods and by Batsto Lake.

Buttonwood Hill is also the closest camping area to Hammonton, the self-proclaimed "Blueberry Capital of the World." New Jersey is responsible for about 20 percent of all blueberries grown in the U.S. Both cranberries and blueberries grow in the Pinelands, and Hammonton has embraced its role as a blueberry production town and celebrates this crop once a year on a Sunday in June at the Red, White, and Blueberry Festival.

Campers interested in less public displays of blueberry appreciation can wander the trails near Buttonwood Hill. Blueberries grow wild in the Pinelands forests and can sometimes be found along the sand trails that wind through the forest near the camping area. Remember not to indiscriminately eat berries and such in the forest.

Buttonwood Hill does not have the same facilities as Atsion or the primitive remote wildness of the canoe-in sites or Batona Camp. But it offers a great combination of privacy, easy road access, economic camping, and proximity to some of the top sites in the Pinelands National Reserve.

WHARTON STATE FOREST: GODFREY BRIDGE CAMPING AREA

WHARTON STATE FOREST'S second most-developed campground has little in common with its first (Atsion) aside from the trees and picnic tables. Atsion is a family campground with a bathhouse and trailer sanitary station. Godfrey Bridge Camping Area, in spite of its $15 per night price tag, might be better compared to the $1 per night primitive wilderness campgrounds that dot this section of the Pinelands. Its vault toilets may not appear to merit the price, but look closer and you will see clearly designated woodland sites, each with a fire ring and picnic table. Many of the peaceful sites are private, with years of undergrowth keeping neighbors from view.

Godfrey Bridge is appealing if you are looking for a secluded forest site, but it also has the advantage of being easily accessed by paved road. Fifteen sites sit around a heart-shaped loop on Godfrey Bridge Road, right after the bridge over the Wading River. These sites are scenic but get the occasional canoe livery shuttle going through the center of camp. The 35 sites in the main camping area get virtually no traffic. Campers who are worried about being miles from the showers at Atsion Recreation Area or Bass River need not worry; the pay-per-shower facility at Wading Pines Camping Resort is only 0.3 miles away. Wading Pines is a private campground that caters mostly to RV and cabin campers, although ten wooded tent sites sit between Wading River and the campground fishing lake. There is a small convenience store at the Wading Pines office where canoes may be rented. Wading Pines has more than 300 sites, 26 rental cabins, recreational facilities, and pets on leashes are allowed. Campers traveling with dogs might consider staying at Wading Pines as dogs are not allowed overnight in New Jersey parks.

At the other end of the tent camping spectrum, featuring no amenities, is Hawkins Bridge Camping

> *The secluded forest si[tes] are appealing, but Godfrey Bridge is als[o] easily accessed by pav[ed] road.*

RATINGS

Beauty: ✫ ✫ ✫ ✫ ✫
Privacy: ✫ ✫ ✫ ✫
Spaciousness: ✫ ✫ ✫ ✫
Quiet: ✫ ✫ ✫ ✫
Security: ✫ ✫ ✫
Cleanliness: ✫ ✫ ✫

ADDRESS: Wharton State Forest
Batsto Office
4110 Nesco Road
Hammonton, NJ
08037

OPERATED BY: State Park Service

INFORMATION: (609) 561-0024

WEB SITE: www.njparksand
forests.org

OPEN: Year-round

SITES: 49

EACH SITE HAS: Picnic table, fire ring

ASSIGNMENT: Choose from
available sites

REGISTRATION: Obtain permit at
Batsto office

FACILITIES: Water, vault toilets

PARKING: At site, 2-vehicle
limit

FEE: $15

ELEVATION: 30 feet

RESTRICTIONS: Pets: Prohibited
Fires: In fire rings
only
Alcohol: Prohibited
Vehicles: Up to 21
feet
Other: Quiet hours
10 p.m.–6 a.m.;
14-night, 6-person,
2-tent limit

Area. From Godfrey Bridge it is only a 1.9-mile drive to Hawkins Bridge, which sits north of Godfrey Bridge in Wharton State Forest along the west branch of the Wading River. The pitted sand access road can be hard on two-wheel-drive sedans, so try to avoid driving to Hawkins Bridge particularly after rainstorms, unless you have a four-wheel-drive vehicle.

Hawkins Bridge is a mostly open, level area dotted with hardwood trees. Outhouses and a water pump are the camp luxuries, and sites are not designated. Campers can put in and take out canoes from Hawkins Bridge, but noncampers are prohibited from using the site and must put canoes in past camp at Tulpehocken Creek. Groups sometimes base themselves at Hawkins Bridge, so look before you camp, or better yet, camp at the family sites back at Godfrey Bridge.

Boat rules are the same at Godfrey Bridge as they are at Hawkins Bridge. Noncampers may not use the ramps for putting canoes into or out of the Wading River. Campers are permitted to use the ramps, although this is only helpful for those who travel with their own canoes or kayaks. Those renting boats must use the access points designated by the local canoe outfitters. The Wading River between Speedwell and Beaver Bridge is one of the easiest, most scenic, and popular canoe routes in New Jersey, and there is no shortage of outfitters ready to supply canoes and transportation. The closest canoe liveries to Godfrey Bridge, in addition to Wading Pines Camping Resort, are Pine Barrens Canoe and Kayak Rental (**www.pinebarrenscanoe.com**) and Mick's Canoe Rental (**www.mickscanoerental.com**), both on CR 563 in Jenkins. Remember that you must plan ahead to camp because both Godfrey Bridge and Hawkins Bridge require camping permits from Batsto office. Popular overnight trips include Oswego Lake or Hawkins Bridge to Bodine Field and Speedwell to Bodine Field or Chips Folly.

Godfrey Bridge and all of the Wharton State Forest camping areas are best known for their access to Pinelands rivers. But plenty of other outdoors recreational activities are available as well. The undeveloped swamps, forests, and floodplains of 1,927-acre

MAP

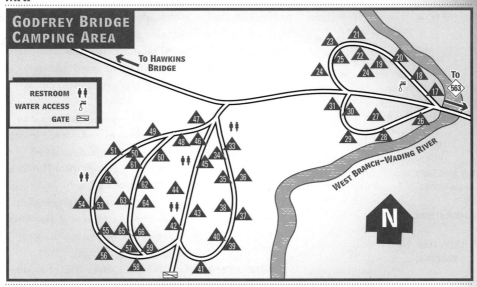

GODFREY BRIDGE CAMPING AREA

To HAWKINS BRIDGE

RESTROOM

WATER ACCESS

GATE

WEST BRANCH–WADING RIVER

To 563

N

Oswego River Natural Area sit directly across CR 563 from Godfrey Bridge Road. The paved roads of the Pinelands National Reserve make great cycling routes, while the unmarked sand paths that wind through Wharton State Forest are open to mountain bikers and hikers. All-terrain vehicles are not permitted in Wharton State Forest, but there are plenty of motor tracks for use by four-wheel-drive vehicles and motorcycles.

Swimming is not permitted in Wading River, but there are guarded swimming areas at Atsion Recreation Area on US 206 and at Lake Absegami in Bass River State Forest. Man-made structures are also present in Wharton State Forest; take a tour of Batsto to view the Pinelands industrial past.

Godfrey Bridge may not have the recreational facilities of Atsion, but its wilderness atmosphere and private setting more than make up for its lack of developed amenities. To some campers, this may even be a strength, making organized-but-simple Godfrey Bridge the most desirable of the Wharton State Forest campgrounds.

GETTING THERE

From the Garden State Parkway, take Exit 67. Turn right onto CR 554 and go 4.3 miles, then head west onto NJ 72 7.8 miles. Turn left onto CR 532 and drive 4 miles. Turn left onto CR 563 and go 8.8 miles to Godfrey Bridge Road. Go right for 1 mile to the campground.

WHARTON STATE FOREST: GOSHEN POND CAMPING AREA

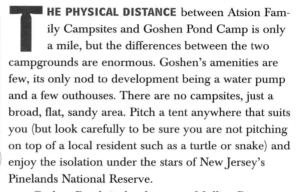

> *The Jersey Devil may live in the nearby woods, but beavers are more common at this primitive camping area.*

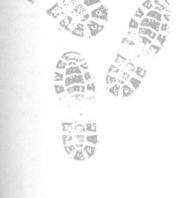

THE PHYSICAL DISTANCE between Atsion Family Campsites and Goshen Pond Camp is only a mile, but the differences between the two campgrounds are enormous. Goshen's amenities are few, its only nod to development being a water pump and a few outhouses. There are no campsites, just a broad, flat, sandy area. Pitch a tent anywhere that suits you (but look carefully to be sure you are not pitching on top of a local resident such as a turtle or snake) and enjoy the isolation under the stars of New Jersey's Pinelands National Reserve.

Goshen Pond sits by the upper Mullica River, along a popular canoe route. It holds a maximum of 200 people and is recommended for horse groups because of its spaciousness and open area. Call ahead to see if any groups have booked the site.

There are outhouses and water pumps on-site but no showers or flushing toilets. Swimming in the Mullica River is prohibited. Campers need not worry, however, about being dirty after a long canoe trip. The bathhouse and beach at Atsion Recreation Area are just a few miles down the road on Atsion Lake. Access fees to the recreation area are $2 for walk-ins and more for cars: parking is $5 on weekdays and $10 on weekends, but is free for cars bearing a current New Jersey State Parks pass. The bathing area is open only during the summer when lifeguards are present. Those looking to work up a sweat before showering can hike the 1-mile trail that loops around the southern bank of Atsion Lake. The recreation area also features picnic facilities, playgrounds, and an activity field.

The closest canoe rental is Adams Canoe Rental (**www.adamscanoerental.com;** phone (609) 268-0189) on Atsion Road. There are many other rental agencies in the Pinelands and most of them offer parking and transportation. From Goshen Pond, try

RATINGS

Beauty: ✪ ✪ ✪ ✪
Privacy: ✪ ✪ ✪
Spaciousness: ✪ ✪ ✪ ✪
Quiet: ✪ ✪ ✪ ✪
Security: ✪ ✪
Cleanliness: ✪ ✪ ✪

canoeing two hours east to the take-out at Atsion Lake. Drive in using a vehicle with four-wheel-drive, if you can, as the dirt-and-sand roads that lead to Goshen Pond can get treacherous after a rain.

As in all New Jersey State camping areas, dogs are prohibited. You'll be glad to have left Fido at home once you read tales of the most famous Pine Barrens resident, the legendary—perhaps fictional—Jersey Devil. Tales of the Jersey Devil have existed in local folklore for hundreds of years.

Legend has it that in 1735 or thereabouts, Mrs. Leeds of a Pine Barrens town (often described as Estellville) discovered that she was pregnant for the thirteenth time. Mrs. Leeds was not rich and had an unhappy marriage. She was less than thrilled with the news of her pregnancy and cursed the child with the statement "Let it be the devil!" In retrospect, perhaps she regretted this remark, as no doubt giving birth to a child with horns, claws, and wings must have been more of a change than she was hoping for.

In some tales, the winged monstrosity turned on its mother and others nearby. In another, it flew up the chimney and out into the forest. In all accounts, the Jersey Devil has been credited with mischief such as raiding chicken coops and slaughtering farm animals. But mostly the creature is known for scaring people with its appearance and its piercing howl, along with its heavy breathing and the hoof prints it leaves behind. When canoeing or hiking, keep an eye peeled for a six- to ten-foot-tall, two-legged, bat-winged reptilian deer with the head of a horse. A clear photo of it might pay for all your Pinelands canoeing trips for the rest of your life.

Russ Juelg of the Pinelands Preservation Alliance holds "Jersey Devil Hunts" a few times a year. Check his Web site, **www.pinelandsalliance.org,** or call the Pinelands Preservation Alliance at (609) 859-8860 for details.

Regardless of whether you participate in an organized hunt or go for it alone, your search for the Jersey Devil is more likely to turn up Jersey Devil T-shirts, coffee mugs, or even a professional hockey team than an actual devil. Local entrepreneurs seem to have

KEY INFORMATION

ADDRESS:	Wharton State Forest Atsion Office 744 US 206 Shamong, NJ 08088
OPERATED BY:	State Park Service
INFORMATION:	(609) 268-0444
WEB SITE:	www.njparks andforests.org
OPEN:	Year-round
SITES:	Open area; maximum 200 people
EACH SITE HAS:	Picnic table, fire ring
ASSIGNMENT:	Choose from available spaces
REGISTRATION:	Obtain permit at either Atsion or Batsto office
FACILITIES:	Water, vault toilets
PARKING:	At site, maximum 2 vehicles
FEE:	$1 per person per night
ELEVATION:	30 feet
RESTRICTIONS:	Pets: Prohibited Fires: Permitted in fire rings only Alcohol: Prohibited Vehicles: 21-foot maximum length Other: Quiet hours 10 p.m.–6 a.m.; 14-night, 6-person, 2-tent limit

MAP

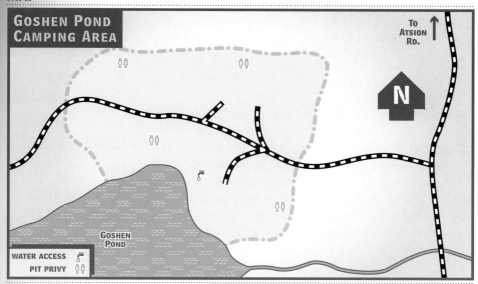

GOSHEN POND CAMPING AREA

TO ATSION RD.

N

GOSHEN POND

WATER ACCESS

PIT PRIVY

GETTING THERE

From the New Jersey Turnpike, take Exit 7 to US 206 south. Drive about 28 miles south on US 206 to Atsion Road. The Atsion Office is at the intersection. Turn right to the campground access road, which is on the left after Atsion Family Campground.

made their own deals with the devil and present his likeness in a variety of money-making schemes.

Odds are the only large creatures you will encounter at Goshen Pond are an animal or another person. So don't let the Jersey Devil scare you away from Wharton State Forest and the Pinelands.

The Pinelands, referred to locally as the Pine Barrens, cover one-fifth of the state of New Jersey. Wharton State Forest is the largest state forest within not just the Pinelands but the entire state. Goshen Pond is one of nine public sites within the park, and of those it presents the best combination of primitive camping near developed recreational activities.

WHARTON STATE FOREST: LOWER FORGE AND MULLICA RIVER CAMPS

LOWER **F**ORGE **C**AMP and Mullica River Camp are inaccessible by design, since motor vehicles of all sorts are prohibited. So bring your horse, your mountain bike, your canoe, or just your own two feet if you want to camp in one of these wilderness sites. Lower Forge has no drinking water, which makes it the less desirable of the two sites to those who don't like to carry their own water. This means campers here are guaranteed a primitive experience with no likelihood of intrusion by neighbors unwilling to rough it.

Distances take on a new meaning when petrol power has no relevance. Lower Forge Camp is a half-mile hike from the nearest road, but the easiest way to get here is to come by canoe, carrying your gear in a waterproof bag. Still, it's no short trek: expect to paddle three hours from Hampton Furnace. The same number of hours will get you and your canoe from Atsion to Mullica River Camp. Set up your tent where you please within the boundaries of either area, and enjoy the rare opportunity to be away from engines of any sort.

Lower Forge Camp sits alongside the Batsto River, while Mullica River Camp is perched next to its namesake. Both the Batsto and Mullica are popular canoe routes with day-trippers. Unmarked sandy roads that lead to river-access points are busy with canoe livery trucks—watch out for traffic if you are hiking and are more than a half-mile from camp, where cars are not prohibited. Advance permits are required for camping here, so there is no danger of day-trippers making impromptu overnight stops.

Both rivers are scenic, easy to paddle, and popular with beginners as well as experienced paddlers. Both can also be navigated by kayak. The Mullica River features open terrain while the Batsto is more varied and even secluded, taking canoeists through cedars. The Mullica River is more easily accessible than the Batsto.

> *Bring your canoe, horse, mountain bike, or your own two feet. Motorized vehicles are not allowed.*

RATINGS

Beauty: ✪ ✪ ✪ ✪
Privacy: ✪ ✪ ✪
Spaciousness: ✪ ✪ ✪ ✪
Quiet: ✪ ✪ ✪ ✪ ✪
Security: ✪ ✪
Cleanliness: ✪ ✪ ✪

KEY INFORMATION

ADDRESS:	Wharton State Forest Atsion Office 744 US 206 Shamong, NJ 08088
OPERATED BY:	State Park Service
INFORMATION:	(609) 268-0444
WEB SITE:	www.njparks andforests.org
OPEN:	Year-round
SITES:	Open areas; Mullica River, 100-person maximum; Lower Forge, 50-person maximum
EACH SITE HAS:	No designated sites
ASSIGNMENT:	Choose from available spaces
REGISTRATION:	Obtain permit at either Atsion or Batsto office
FACILITIES:	Water at Mullica River, vault toilets at both
PARKING:	Park at designated lots and hike in
FEE:	$2 per person per night
ELEVATION:	40 feet
RESTRICTIONS:	**Pets:** Prohibited **Fires:** Prohibited **Alcohol:** Prohibited **Vehicles:** Prohibited **Other:** Canoe-in or hike-in only; no vehicle access; horses permitted

Adams Canoe Rental (**www.adamscanoerental.com**; phone (609) 268-0189) and Bel Haven Canoe (**www.belhavencanoe.com**; phone (609) 965-2205) service this section of Wharton State Forest.

Hikers are also well served in this part of the Pinelands National Reserve. The flat, accessible 50-mile Batona Trail that traverses the forest from Brendan T. Byrne State Forest to Bass River State Forest passes at its halfway point just south of Lower Forge Camp. No horses or mountain bikes are permitted on Batona Trail except where it follows existing roads. Those preferring a shorter hike can hike from Atsion to Lower Forge via Springer's Brook and the railroad, for a total distance of 7.9 miles.

The 9-mile Mullica River Trail parallels the Mullica River, connecting Atsion and Batsto. The Mullica River campground is in the middle, 4 miles from Batsto and 5 miles from Atsion. Keep your eyes open for deer, beaver, and birds. The trail passes through wetlands and under pine and cedar trees. From Batsto to Constable Bridge, be alert for trucks towing canoes. You'll pass several appealing beaches as you hike along the Mullica; however, remember that swimming is not permitted.

Both rivers and the Mullica River Trail pass through Batsto Natural Area, a 10,000-acre area reserved for forest communities that border the Mullica and Batsto Rivers. With its savannas, open marshes, dry soil, and tea-colored rivers, the Batsto Natural Area is the Pinelands National Reserve in miniature.

Immediately south of Batsto Natural Area is the once-industrial, now-historic Batsto Village. For 100 years, Batsto Village thrived through various industrial trends. First, it was the site of an iron furnace. Bog iron is a naturally occurring form of iron that can be dug out of the Pinelands. After the decline of the iron industry, Batsto became the site of a glass-production operation: the iron-rich soil of the Pine Barrens also features an ideal combination of sand and water, ideal for making glass. Joseph Wharton, a businessman from Philadelphia, purchased Batsto in 1876. He continued buying surrounding lands and at the time of his death

MAP

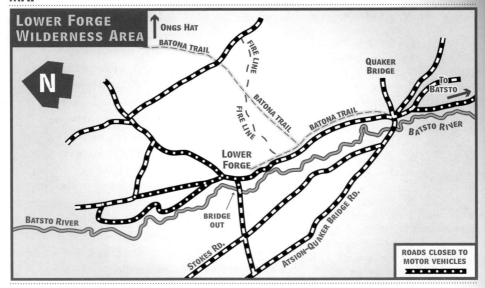

LOWER FORGE WILDERNESS AREA

↑ ONGS HAT

BATONA TRAIL

FIRE LINE

QUAKER BRIDGE

TO BATSTO →

N

BATONA TRAIL

FIRE LINE

BATONA TRAIL

BATSTO RIVER

LOWER FORGE

BATSTO RIVER

BRIDGE OUT

STOKES RD.

ATSION-QUAKER BRIDGE RD.

ROADS CLOSED TO MOTOR VEHICLES

in 1909 owned 96,000 acres of southern Jersey. Fortunately for the population of New Jersey, Wharton's plan to utilize the pristine watershed in a money-making endeavor did not come to fruition. Instead (perhaps inadvertently), Wharton became an early conservationist, preserving the area's wilderness and its fragile watershed for future generations.

The State of New Jersey acquired Wharton's land in the 1950s, adding to it another 15,000 acres over the years. Today, Wharton State Forest is the largest forest in the New Jersey State Park system, stretching from near the Jersey shore to Philadelphia. Lower Forge Camp and Mullica River Camp are the only two sites in the system that are not accessible by motorized vehicle, and that makes them unique treasures in this unusual natural environment.

GETTING THERE

From the New Jersey Turnpike, take Exit 7 to US 206 south. Drive about 28 miles south on US 206 to Atsion Road. The office is at the intersection. From the office, take the dirt road on the left (Quaker Bridge Road). After 2.5 miles, turn right onto the 3-mile road to the Mullica River parking area. Lower Forge parking area is another 1.7 miles to the left. Hike 0.5 miles to access the Lower Forge Campground.

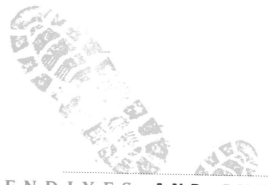

APPENDIXES **AND** INDEX

APPENDIX A
CAMPING EQUIPMENT
CHECKLIST

Except for the large and bulky items on this list, I keep a plastic storage container full of the essentials for car camping so they're ready to go when I am. I make a last-minute check of the inventory, resupply anything that's low or missing, and away I go.

COOKING UTENSILS
Bottle opener
Bottles of salt, pepper, spices, sugar, cooking oil, and maple syrup in water-proof, spillproof containers
Can opener
Corkscrew
Cups, plastic or tin
Dish soap (biodegradable), sponge, and towel
Fire starter
Flatware
Food of your choice
Frying pan, spatula
Fuel for stove
Lighter, matches in waterproof container
Plates
Pocketknife
Pot with lid
Stove
Tin foil
Wooden spoon

FIRST–AID KIT
Aspirin
Band-Aids
First-aid cream
Gauze pads
Insect repellent
Moleskin
Sunscreen/chapstick
Tape, waterproof adhesive

SLEEPING GEAR
Pillow
Sleeping bag
Sleeping pad, inflatable or insulated
Tent with ground tarp and rainfly

MISCELLANEOUS
Bath soap (biodegradable), wash cloth, and towel
Camp chair
Candles
Cooler
Deck of cards
Flashlight/headlamp
Paper towels
Plastic zip-top bags
Sunglasses
Toilet paper
Water bottle
Wool blanket

OPTIONAL
Barbecue grill
Binoculars
Field guides on bird, plant, and wildlife identification
Fishing rod and tackle
Lantern
Maps (road, trail, topographic, etc.)

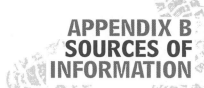

APPENDIX B
SOURCES OF
INFORMATION

Appalachian Trail Conference
www.appalachiantrail.org

Genovese, Peter. *New Jersey Curiosities: Quirky Characters, Roadside Oddities, and Other Offbeat Stuff.* Globe Pequot Press, 2003.

Lurie, Maxine N. and Marc Mappen, editors. *Encyclopedia of New Jersey.* Rutgers University Press, 2004.

New Jersey Campground Owner's Association
www.newjerseycampgrounds.com

New Jersey Coastal Heritage Trail Route
www.nps.gov/neje

New Jersey State Parks, Forests, and Historic Sites
www.njparksandforests.com

New York–New Jersey Trail Conference
www.nynjtc.org

Parnes, Robert. *Paddling the Jersey Pine Barrens.* Falcon, 2002.

Sceurman, Mark and Mark Moran. *Weird N.J.: Your Travel Guide to New Jersey's Local Legends and Best Kept Secrets.* Barnes and Noble, 2003.

Scofield, Bruce and Stella Green and H. Neil Zimmerman. *50 Hikes in New Jersey.* Countryman Press, 1997.

Brown, Michael P. *New Jersey Parks, Forest, and Natural Areas: A Guide.* Rutgers University Press, 1997.

Doo Wop Preservation League, Wildwood, NJ
www.doowopusa.org

Fernicola, Richard G. *Twelve Days of Terror: A Definitive Investigation of the 1916 New Jersey Shark Attacks.* The Lyons Press, 2001.

McPhee, John. *The Pine Barrens.* Farar, Straus & Giroux, 1978.

New Jersey Audubon Society
www.njaudubon.org

New Jersey's Great Northwest Skylands
www.njskylands.com

New Jersey Pinelands National Reserve (National Park Service)
www.nps.gov/pine

Roadside America: Your Online Guide to Offbeat Attractions (NJ section)
www.roadsideamerica.com

Scheller, William G. and Kay. *New Jersey Off the Beaten Path: A Guide to Unique Places.* Globe Pequot Press, 2002.

Westergaard, Barbara. *New Jersey: A Guide to the State.* Rutgers University Press, 1998.

INDEX

A

Absegami Natural Area, 98
Albocondo Campground, 112–113
alcohol, 26
Aldrin, Buzz, 90
Allaire, James P., 62
Allaire State Park, 62–64
Allamuchy Mountain State Park, 44
American Revolution
  Hancock House Historic Site, 131
  Monmouth Battlefield State Park, 87
  Red Bank Plantation, 142
  tea protests, monument, 130
  Washington Crossing State Park, 66
Annie M. Carter Interpretive Center, Batsto Lake,
  154
Appalachian National Scenic Trail (A.T.)
  Delaware Water Gap, 28
  High Point State Park access, 35
  Stokes State Forest access, 49, 53
  Worthington State Forest, 58–59
  Yards Creek access, 24
Arbuckel, George, 140
archery, Campgaw Mountain, 9
astronomy
  Jenny Jump Observatory, 38
  New Jersey Astronomical Association
    Observatory, 90
  Paul H. Robinson Observatory, 90
  United Astronomy Clubs observatory, 84
Atlantic City, 95
Atlantic City North Family Campground, 94–96
Atlantic County Park at Estell Manor, 120–122
Atlantic County Park at Lake Lenape, 123–125
Atlantic County Rowing Association, 123
Atsion Lake, 144, 145
Atsion Recreation Area, 144–146, 152, 159
Audubon Society, 17

B

Back to Nature Trail. *See* Batona Trail
Barnegat Bay Sail Charters, 104
Barnegat Lighthouse State Park, 104, 116
Bass River State Forest, 94, 97–99, 116
Batona Trail
  Bass River State Forest, 98
  Brendan T. Byrne State Forest, 133
  Lower Forge Camp, Wharton State Forest, 163
  Pinelands, 94–95

  Timberline Lake Camping Resort, 116
  Wharton State Forest, 147–148
Batsto Lake, 154
Batsto Natural Area, 151–152, 163
Batsto River, 162
Batsto Village, 153–154, 163
bears, 4
beauty, campground rating system, 3
Beaver Branch Canoe Landing, Wading River, 150
Beaver Hill Campground, 32
Belleplain State Forest
  hiking trails in, 136–137
  Meisle Field and CCC Camp, 126–128
Benjamin Franklin National Memorial, 142
Bergen County, 11–13, 14
Berkeley Island County Park, 105
Bethlehem Loading Company, 121
bicycling, Harrisville Lake to Evans Bridge loop, 151
Big Flatbrook River, 46–48
Birch Grove Park, 95, 100–102
black bears, 4
Blairstown, 57
Blue Mine Falls, 18
Blue Mountain Lake, 29
Blue Mountain Trail, 46
blueberry production, 154
Bodine Field Camp, Wharton State Forest, 150–152
Brendan T. Byrne State Forest, 132–134, 147
Brendan T. Byrne State Park, 98
Brotzmanville, 60
Bull's Island Recreation Area, 65–67
Buttermilk Falls, 47
Buttonwood Hill Camp, Wharton State Forest,
  153–155
Byrne, Governor, 134

C

Camp Acagisca, 123, 124
Camp Glen Gray campground, 11–13
Camp Taylor, 22–24
Campgaw Mountain, 8–10, 15
campgrounds
  See also featured sites
  locator map, viii
  rating system for, 2–4
canoeing
  Batsto River, 162–163
  Cedar Creek Campground, 103
  Delaware River, 25, 66, 71–72

canoeing *(continued)*
    Goshen Pond Camping Area, 159–160
    Lake Lenape, 124
    Manasquan River, 64, 86–87
    Wharton State Forest, Atsion Lake, 145
    Wharton State Forest, Bodine Field, 150
Cape May Lighthouse, 127
Cape May Migratory Bird Observatory, 127
Cape May Migratory Bird Refuge, 107
Cape May Point State Park, 107, 127
Carranza, Captain Emilio, 148
Carranza Memorial, 147–148
CCC/Forest Fire Service Memorial, Bass River, 98
Cedar Creek, 111
Cedar Creek Campground, 103–105
Cedar Swamp Natural Area, 35, 133
Central Region of New Jersey, 61–91
Checker, Chubby, 107
Cheesequake State Park, 68–70
Chikahoki Falls, 18
Civilian Conservation Corps (CCC), 90, 97, 126, 138
cleanliness, campground rating system, 4
Clinton Wildlife Management Area, 77
Coastal Heritage Trail, Corson's Inlet, 102
cooking, protecting food from animals, 4
Corson's Inlet, 101
Corson's Inlet State Park, 136
Cowtown Rodeo, 140
Cox, John, 154
cranberry bogs, 132–133
Crater Lake, 29
Crowley Landing, Mullica River, 153
cycling, Harrisville Lake to Evans Bridge loop, 151

D
Darlington County Park, 9, 15
Daynor, George, 140
deer ticks, 5
Delaware and Raritan Canal, 43, 65
Delaware River, 25, 26, 41, 47, 65, 141
Delaware River Family Campground, 71–73
Delaware Water Gap National Recreational Area, 22, 23
    canoe-in, 25–27
    hike-in, 28–30
Delsea Region, 130, 131, 143
Depew Island, 26
Dingmans Ferry, 26
dogs
    at Harmony Ridge Campground, 31
    in New Jersey state parks, 94
    North Wildwood Camping Resort, 106
Doo-Wop Preservation League, 107
Double Trouble State Park, 103–104, 111
Dover Township Parks Department, 109
Dryden Kuser National Area, 35
Duck Pond, Swartswood State Park, 56
Dunnfield Creek, 59

E
Edgar Felix Bicycle Path, 63
Edwin B. Forsythe National Wildlife Refuge, 95, 117
Edwin E. Aldrin Astronomical Center, 90
endangered species, 152
Estell Manor, Atlantic County Park at, 120–122, 125
Estellville Glassworks, 121–122

F
Faery Hole (cave), 38
fishing
    Birch Grove Park, 101
    Delaware and Raritan Canal State Park, 66
    Delaware River, 59
    Lake Absegami, 99
    Lake Nummy, 127
    Parvin, Thundergust Lakes, 139
    Ramapo River, 14
    Round Valley Reservoir, 76
    Swartswood Lake, 56
    Toms River, 110, 112
food, protecting from animals, 4
Fort Mott, 131
Fort Mott State Park, 143
Fox Nature Center, Atlantic County Park, 121
Franklin, Benjamin, 1, 142
Franklin Lakes, 9
French and Indian Wars, 57
Frog Pond, Swartswood State Park, 56
Frontier Campground, 135–137

G
garbage disposal, 4–5
Garden State Parkway, 107
Ghost Lake, 37, 38
Gloucester County, Greenwich Lake Park, 141–142
Godfrey Bridge Camping Area, Wharton State Forest, 156–158
Golden Pond, Birch Grove Park, 100
golf, Spring Meadow Golf Course, Allaire, 63
Greater Wildwoods Tourism Authority, 107
Green Bank, 151
Greenwich Lake Park, 141–142
Greenwich Tea Burning Monument, 130

H
Hacklebarney State Park, 89
Hammonton, 154
Hancock House Historic Site, 131
Harmony Ridge Campground, 31–33
Harrisville Ruins, 151
Hawkins Bridge Camping Area, 156–157
Headley Overlook, 41
Heislerville horseshoe crab spawning, 131
Hereford Inlet Lighthouse, 136
Hewitt-Butler Trails, 18
High Bridge, 91
High Point Cross Country Ski Center, 36
High Point Monument, 35
High Point State Park, 30, 32, 34–36

Highlands Trail, 18, 41, 44, 78
Hooks Creek Lake, 69
horseshoe crab spawning, Heislerville, 131
Howell Iron Works Company, 62
Hudson River, 41
Hunterdon County, 79, 80

I

insects, repellants, 4–5
Island Beach State Park, 104, 111, 113

J

Jaggers Point Campground, Parvin State Park, 138
James, Brenda, 84
Jenny Jump State Forest, 37–39
Jersey Devil, 147, 160
Jersey Shore, 136
Juelg, Russ, 147, 160

K

Kalmyck Republic, 138
kayaking. See canoeing
Keen's Grist Mill, Swartswood Lake, 56
Kittatinny Glacial Geology Trail, 50
Kittatinny Mountains, 22, 25, 28, 58, 85

L

Lake Absegami, 97–98, 152, 157
Lake Hopatcong, 40
Lake Lenape, 120, 123–125
Lake Marcia, 34, 35
Lake Nummy, 126, 127, 129, 130, 137
Lake Ocquittunk, 53
Lake Ocquittunk Camping Area, 46–48
Lakota Wolf Preserve, 22, 84
Lebanon Glass Works, 132
Lebanon State Forest, 134
Leeds, Mrs., 160
legend to maps, ix
Lenape Indians, 25, 38, 44, 45, 70
Lenni Lenape Indians, 70, 126, 145
Liberty State Park, 65
Little Swartswood Lake, 55
Long Beach Island, 95, 97, 104, 116
Lower Forge Camp, Wharton State Forest, 162–164
Lucy the Elephant, Margate, 102
Lyme disease, 5

M

Mahlon Dickerson Reservation, 40–42
Manasquan River, 64, 86–87
maps
   See also featured sites
   legend to, ix
   New Jersey campground locator, viii
   New Jersey key, vii
Matawan Creek, 69
Meisle Field, Belleplain State Forest, 126–128
missile site at Riker Hill Park, 9
Monmouth Battlefield State Park, 87
Monroe, Dr. Will S., 18

Montclair State University, 52
Morris Canal, 43, 65
Morris County Park System, 40–41
Mount Lake, 38
Mount Minsi, 72
Mount Misery, 133
Mount Tammany, 23, 59, 72
Mountain Farm, Teetertown, 81–82
Mullica River, 153, 159, 162–164
Musconetcong River, 43, 45

N

National Park Service, 28
Native Americans
   Lenape Indians, 25, 38, 44, 45, 70
   Lenni Lenape Indians, 70, 126, 145
New Jersey
   camping generally, 2
   Central Region, 61–91
   maps key, vii
   Northern Region, 7–19
   Shore Region, 93–117
   Southern Region, 119–164
   Western Region, 21–60
New Jersey Astronomical Association Observatory, 89
New Jersey (battleship), 143
New Jersey Coastal Heritage Trail, 95, 104, 130, 136, 143
New Jersey School of Conservation, 52
New Jersey State Aquarium, 141, 142–143
New Jersey State Park Service, 28
Newark Watershed, 18
Nike Battery NY-93/43, 9
noise, campground rating system, 3
Nomoco Activity Area, Triple Brook, 86
North Branch, Toms River, 109
North Wildwood Camping Resort, 106–108
Northern Region of New Jersey, 7–19
Northfield Garden Club, Birch Grove Park, 100
Norvin Green State Forest, 18
Noyes Museum of Art, Oceanville, 96

O

observatories
   Jenny Jump Observatory, 38
   New Jersey Astronomical Association Observatory, 89
   Paul H. Robinson Observatory, 90
   United Astronomy Clubs observatory, 84
Ocean City, 101, 136
Oswego River Natural Area, 151, 157
Otter Hole, 18

P

Palace Depression, the, 140
Parker Brook, 53
parking, New Jersey State Park annual passes, 144
Parvin State Park, 138–140
Paul H. Robinson Observatory, 90

Pequest Trout Hatchery, 84
Peters Valley Craft Education Center, 47
pets in camping areas, 4
Pine Barrens, 147
Pine Barrens River Ramble bike route, 151
Pine Creek Railroad, 63
Pinelands, 86, 161
Pinelands National Reserve, 94, 113, 147, 154
Pinelands Preservation Alliance (PPA), 147
Pitcher, Molly, 87
PNC Bank Arts Center, 68
Port Jervis, 34
Port Murray, 81
Prallsville Mills, 66
privacy, campground rating system, 3
Pygmy Pines, Bass River State Forest, 99

Q
quiet, campground rating system, 3

R
Ramapo Valley County Reservation, 11–13, 14–16
Raritan Canal, 43
Raritan Canal State Park, 65
Raritan River, 79
rating system for campgrounds, 2–4
Read, Charles, 153–154
Red Bank Plantation, Battlefield Park, 142
repellant, insect, 5
Revolutionary War
    Hancock House Historic Site, 131
    Monmouth Battlefield State Park, 87
    Red Bank Battlefield Park, 142
    tea protests, monument, 130
    Washington Crossing State Park, 66
Richards, William, 154
Riker Hill Park, 9
Ringwood State Park, 15
Risdon, Ed and Doris Ann, 32
Riverwood Park, 109–111
Round Valley Recreation Area, 74–76, 89

S
Saddle Ridge Horseback Riding Center, 9
Saffin Pond Area, 41, 42
Sandy Hook, Cheesequake State Park, 69
Sawmill Lake, 34, 36
Saxton Falls, 44
Saxton Falls Dam, 45
Scarlet Oak Pond, 14
scuba diving, 75
Seaside Heights, 110, 113
security, campground rating system, 3
Ship Bottom Beach, Long Beach Island, 95
Shore Region of New Jersey, 93–117
Shotwell Camping Area, Stokes State Forest, 49–51
Sinatra, Frank, 1
Six Flags Great Adventure theme park, 87, 110,
    112–113

snakes, 4
Somers Brick Yard, 100
South River, 120, 122
Southern Region of New Jersey, 119–164
Space Farms Zoo, 23
spaciousness, campground rating system, 3
Spring Lake, 88
Spring Lake, Swartswood State Park, 56
Spring Meadow Golf Course, Allaire, 63
Spruce Run Recreation Area, 77–79
Spruce Run Reservoir, 77–78
Stalin, Joseph, 138
star rating system for campgrounds, 2–4
stargazing. *See* astronomy
Statue of Liberty, Vineland, 139–140
Steenykill Lake, 34
Stephen's Creek, 122
Stephens State Park, 43–45
Stokes, Edward C., 49
Stokes State Forest, 28, 30, 31, 32, 46–54
Stone Harbor Bird Sanctuary, 108
Stone Harbor, Wetlands Institute, 108, 136
Stony Lake, 51, 53
Stow Creek Viewing Area, Delsea Region, 131
Strathmere Natural Area, 101
Stump Creek, 68
Sunfish Pond, Worthington State Forest, 59
Sunrise Mountain, 32, 49–50
Surf and Stream Campground, 110, 112–114
Sussex County, 50
Swamp Trail Boardwalk, Atlantic County Park,
    120–121
Swartswood, Captain Anthony, 57
Swartswood State Park, 55–57

T
tea protests, American Revolution, 130
Teetertown Ravine Nature Preserve, 80–82
tent burglary, 15–16
Thundergust Lake, 138
ticks, 4–5
Tillman Brook, 47
Tillman Ravine, 33, 47
Timberlane Campground, 141–143
Timberline Lake Camping Resort, 115–117
Tocks Island Dam, 27
Toms River, 109
treefrog, endangered, 152
Triple Brook Camping Resort, 83–85
Tuckerton Seaport, 96

U
United Astronomy Clubs observatory, 84

V
Valley Forge, 141
Vineland, 139
Voorhees, Gov. Foster M., 89
Voorhees State Park, 89–91

W

Wading Pines Camping Resort, 156
Wading River, 150, 152, 156–158
Wanaque Reservoir, 18
War of 1812, Wharton State Forest, 145
Warren E. Fox Nature Center, Atlantic County
    Park, 121
Washington Crossing State Park, 66
Washington, George, 87
Washington Lake Park, Sewell, 142
Waterloo Village, 43, 44
Weir Dam, 66
Weird N.J. (Sceurman and Moran), 38
Weis Ecology Center, 17–19
Weis, Walter and May, 18
West Pine Plains Natural Area, 99
Western Region of New Jersey, 21–60
Wetlands Institute, Stone Harbor, 108, 136
Weymouth Park, 125
Wharton, Joseph, 145–146, 151, 154, 163–164

Wharton State Forest
    Atsion, 144–146
    Batona Camp, 147–149
    Bodine Field Camp, 150–152
    Buttonwoood Hill Camp, 153–155
    Godfrey Bridge Camping Area, 156–158
    Goshen Pond Camping Area, 159–161
    Lower Forge, Mullica River Camps, 162–164
Whitall House, Red Bank Plantation, 142
Whitesbog Village, 132–133
William J. Dudley Park, 105
Willoughby Brook, Voorhees State Park, 90
Winding River Park, 110
wolves, 22–23
Worthington, Charles, 60
Worthington State Forest, 25, 26, 28, 29, 58–60
Wyanokie Trails, 18

Y

Yards Creek, 24

ABOUT THE AUTHOR

ORIGINALLY FROM Northern Virginia, Marie Javins as a child was dragged all over the Shenandoah Valley and surrounding mountains. Back then she hated camping, fishing, and looking at wildlife, and after college immediately moved to New York City. She did not learn to love camping again until, as an adult, she camped around Africa as a matter of financial necessity. Since then she has tent-camped her way across the United States and New Zealand.

Marie was an editor and colorist for Marvel Comics for 13 years before taking up travel writing. She currently lives in downtown Jersey City, New Jersey, where she is authoring *Slow Boat to Everywhere,* a book about her trip around the world by surface transport (for more details, go to **www.MariesWorldTour.com**).